T0155614

METHODS IN MOLECULAR BIOLOGY

Series Editor
John M. Walker
School of Life and Medical Sciences
University of Hertfordshire
Hatfield, Hertfordshire, AL10 9AB, UK

For further volumes:
http://www.springer.com/series/7651

Circular RNAs

Methods and Protocols

Edited by

Christoph Dieterich

Department of Internal Medicine III, Klaus Tschira Institute for Integrative Computational Cardiology, University Hospital Heidelberg, Heidelberg, Germany

Argyris Papantonis

Center for Molecular Medicine Cologne (CMMC), University of Cologne, Cologne, Germany

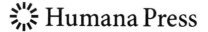 Humana Press

Editors
Christoph Dieterich
Department of Internal Medicine III
Klaus Tschira Institute for Integrative
Computational Cardiology
University Hospital Heidelberg
Heidelberg, Germany

Argyris Papantonis
Center for Molecular Medicine Cologne
(CMMC)
University of Cologne
Cologne, Germany

ISSN 1064-3745   ISSN 1940-6029   (electronic)
Methods in Molecular Biology
ISBN 978-1-4939-8521-0   ISBN 978-1-4939-7562-4   (eBook)
https://doi.org/10.1007/978-1-4939-7562-4

Printed on acid-free paper

This Humana Press imprint is published by Springer Nature
The registered company is Springer Science+Business Media, LLC
The registered company address is: 233 Spring Street, New York, NY 10013, U.S.A.

Preface

Although isolated examples of circularized RNA molecules were already described more than 20 years ago [1, 2], it was not until quite recently that the prevalence of circular RNAs (circRNAs) was revealed. The advent of massively parallel sequencing technology allowed researchers to catalogue circRNAs across eukaryotic and prokaryotic systems (e.g., [3–7]). Their surprisingly high titers within cells are a result of (1) their circular form that renders them far less susceptible to degradation by exoribonucleases, and (2) their multiple regions of origin. circRNAs originate from thousands of different genes active per cell type (both protein-coding and noncoding), and the final circular RNA molecule may include exonic, intronic, or exonic and intronic sequences [8].

Despite their abundance, the functions served by circRNAs remain largely enigmatic, and it is has been suggested that many of them might rather be long-lived transcriptional by-products [9]. To date, mainly three types of functions have been described. First, their role as potent miRNA sponges: ciRS-7 constitutes a prime example, carrying >70 recognition sites for human miR-7, thus sequestering this miRNA from intracellular circulation [10, 11], while circHIPK3 acts as a sponge of multiple miRNAs [12]. Nonetheless, only very few circRNAs are predicted to be able to carry out such a "sponging" activity. Second, their role as (post-) transcriptional regulators: For example, particular exon-intron circRNAs have been described that can regulate the expression levels of their parental genes via RNA-RNA interactions (which may also involve the U1 snRNA; [13]), via direct competition with pre-mRNA splicing [9, 14], or even by modulation of transcription factor activity [15, 16]. Finally, there exist circRNAs with a role in translation: circRNAs were shown to be translationally competent and to carry short open reading frames [17, 18]; hence, three recent studies exemplifying their translatability greatly expand the coding and regulatory eukaryotic landscape [15, 16, 19, 20]. Although not a functional aspect *per se*, one should also note here that circRNAs show significant potential as biomarkers, for example in tissue aging [21, 22] and in cancer [13, 23].

CircRNA expression is cell type- and tissue-specific and can be largely independent of the expression level of the linear host gene. Thus, regulation of expression might be an important aspect with regard to control of circular RNA function. Initial evidence suggests that circular RNA biogenesis proceeds through RNA hairpin intermediates, which are modulated by RNA modifications (e.g., A->I editing at flanking inverted repeats; [24]) and/or RNA-binding proteins (e.g., QKI; [25]). Conceptually, RNA structure shapes in such a way that the downstream 5' splice site is close to a 3' upstream splice site [26]. This facilitates a back-splicing event leading to a circularized RNA molecule with different covalent configurations: 3'–5' linkages, containing only exonic sequence; 2'–5' linkages (intronic lariats); or 3'–5' linkages that contain retained intronic sequences [27]. There is an active discussion whether circular RNAs predominantly emerge from direct back-splicing or exon skipping events [9].

Taken together, circRNAs still comprise unexplored territory as regards many of their basic biogenesis mechanisms and functional implications. The molecular and bioinformatics toolkit for studying circRNAs is continuously expanding, and the present volume aims at providing access to well-established approaches for identifying, characterizing, and manipulating circRNAs in vitro, in vivo, and in silico—and in doing so this compilation of 17 chapters also highlights the breakthroughs and the challenges in this new field of research.

Heidelberg, Germany   *Christoph Dieterich*
Cologne, Germany   *Argyris Papantonis*

References

1. Capel B, Swain A, Nicolis S, Hacker A, Walter M, Koopman P, Goodfellow P, Lovell-Badge R (1993) Circular transcripts of the testis-determining gene Sry in adult mouse testis. Cell 73:1019–1030

2. Nigro JM, Cho KR, Fearon ER, Kern SE, Ruppert JM, Oliner JD, Kinzler KW, Vogelstein B (1991) Scrambled exons. Cell 64:607–613

3. Danan M, Schwartz S, Edelheit S, Sorek R (2012) Transcriptome-wide discovery of circular RNAs in Archaea. Nucleic Acids Res 40:3131–3142

4. Dong R, Ma XK, Chen LL, Yang L (2016) Increased complexity of circRNA expression during species evolution. RNA Biol 16:1–11

5. Sun X, Wang L, Ding J, Wang Y, Wang J, Zhang X, Che Y, Liu Z, Zhang X, Ye J, Wang J, Sablok G, Deng Z, Zhao H (2016) Integrative analysis of Arabidopsis thaliana transcriptomics reveals intuitive splicing mechanism for circular RNA. FEBS Lett 590:3510–3516

6. Wang PL, Bao Y, Yee MC, Barrett SP, Hogan GJ, Olsen MN, Dinneny JR, Brown PO, Salzman J (2014) Circular RNA is expressed across the eukaryotic tree of life. PLoS One 9:e90859

7. Xu S, Xiao S, Qiu C, Wang Z (2017) Transcriptome-wide identification and functional investigation of circular RNA in the teleost large yellow croaker (*Larimichthys crocea*). Mar Genomics 32:71–78

8. Meng X, Li X, Zhang P, Wang J, Zhou Y, Chen M (2017) Circular RNA: an emerging key player in RNA world. Brief Bioinform 18:547–557

9. Kelly S, Greenman C, Cook PR, Papantonis A (2015) Exon skipping is correlated with exon circularization. J Mol Biol 427:2414–2417

10. Hansen TB, Jensen TI, Clausen BH, Bramsen JB, Finsen B, Damgaard CK, Kjems J (2013) Natural RNA circles function as efficient microRNA sponges. Nature 495:384–388

11. Memczak S, Jens M, Elefsinioti A, Torti F, Krueger J, Rybak A, Maier L, Mackowiak SD, Gregersen LH, Munschauer M, Loewer A, Ziebold U, Landthaler M, Kocks C, le Noble F, Rajewsky N (2013) Circular RNAs are a large class of animal RNAs with regulatory potency. Nature 495:333–338

12. Zheng Q, Bao C, Guo W, Li S, Chen J, Chen B, Luo Y, Lyu D, Li Y, Shi G, Liang L, Gu J, He X, Huang S (2016) Circular RNA profiling reveals an abundant circHIPK3 that regulates cell growth by sponging multiple miRNAs. Nat Commun 7:11215

13. Li Z, Huang C, Bao C, Chen L, Lin M, Wang X, Zhong G, Yu B, Hu W, Dai L, Zhu P, Chang Z, Wu Q, Zhao Y, Jia Y, Xu P, Liu H, Shan G (2015) Exon-intron circular RNAs regulate transcription in the nucleus. Nat Struct Mol Biol 22:256–264

14. Ashwal-Fluss R, Meyer M, Pamudurti NR, Ivanov A, Bartok O, Hanan M, Evantal N, Memczak S, Rajewsky N, Kadener S (2014) circRNA biogenesis competes with pre-mRNA splicing. Mol Cell 56:55–66

15. Yang Q, WW D, Wu N, Yang W, Awan FM, Fang L, Ma J, Li X, Zeng Y, Yang Z, Dong J, Khorshidi A, Yang BB (2017a) A circular RNA promotes tumorigenesis by inducing c-myc nuclear translocation. Cell Death Differ 24:1609–1620

16. Yang Y, Fan X, Mao M, Song X, Wu P, Zhang Y, Jin Y, Yang Y, Chen LL, Wang Y, Wong CC, Xiao X, Wang Z (2017b) Extensive translation of circular RNAs driven by N(6)-methyladenosine. Cell Res 27:626–641

17. Abe N, Matsumoto K, Nishihara M, Nakano Y, Shibata A, Maruyama H, Shuto S, Matsuda A, Yoshida M, Ito Y, Abe H (2015) Rolling circle translation of circular RNA in living human cells. Sci Rep 5:16435

18. Wang Y, Wang Z (2015) Efficient backsplicing produces translatable circular mRNAs. RNA 21:172–179

19. Legnini I, Di Timoteo G, Rossi F, Morlando M, Briganti F, Sthandier O, Fatica A, Santini T, Andronache A, Wade M, Laneve P, Rajewsky N, Bozzoni I (2017) Circ-ZNF609 is a circular RNA that can be translated and functions in myogenesis. Mol Cell 66:22–37

20. Pamudurti NR, Bartok O, Jens M, Ashwal-Fluss R, Stottmeister C, Ruhe L, Hanan M, Wyler E, Perez-Hernandez D, Ramberger E, Shenzis S, Samson M, Dittmar G, Landthaler M, Chekulaeva M, Rajewsky N, Kadener S (2017) Translation of circRNAs. Mol Cell 66:9–21

21. Gruner H, Cortés-López M, Cooper DA, Bauer M, Miura P (2016) CircRNA accumulation in the aging mouse brain. Sci Rep 6:38907

22. Westholm JO, Miura P, Olson S, Shenker S, Joseph B, Sanfilippo P, Celniker SE, Graveley BR, Lai EC (2014) Genome-wide analysis of drosophila circular RNAs reveals their structural and sequence properties and age-dependent neural accumulation. Cell Rep 9(5):1966–1980

23. Ahmed I, Karedath T, Andrews SS, Al-Azwani IK, Mohamoud YA, Querleu D, Rafii A, Malek JA (2016) Altered expression pattern of circular RNAs in primary and metastatic sites of epithelial ovarian carcinoma. Oncotarget 7(24):36366–36381

24. Ivanov A, Memczak S, Wyler E, Torti F, Porath HT, Orejuela MR, Piechotta M, Levanon EY, Landthaler M, Dieterich C, Rajewsky N (2015) Analysis of intron sequences reveals hallmarks of circular RNA biogenesis in animals. Cell Rep 10:170–177

25. Conn SJ, Pillman KA, Toubia J, Conn VM, Salmanidis M, Phillips CA, Roslan S, Schreiber AW, Gregory PA, Goodall GJ (2015) The RNA binding protein quaking regulates formation of circRNAs. Cell 160:1125–1134

26. Zhang XO, Wang HB, Zhang Y, Lu X, Chen LL, Yang L (2014) Complementary sequence-mediated exon circularization. Cell 159:134–147

27. Salzman J (2016) Circular RNA expression: its potential regulation and function. Trends Genet 32:309–316

Contents

Contributors

KOTB ABDELMOHSEN • *Laboratory of Genetics and Genomics, National Institute on Aging-Intramural Research Program, National Institutes of Health, Baltimore, MD, USA*

HIROSHI ABE • *Department of Chemistry, Graduate School of Science, Nagoya University, Nagoya, Japan*

NAOKO ABE • *Department of Chemistry, Graduate School of Science, Nagoya University, Nagoya, Japan*

DENIZ BARTSCH • *Cologne Excellence Cluster on Cellular Stress Responses in Aging-Associated Diseases, University of Cologne, Cologne, Germany; Institute for Neurophysiology, University of Cologne, Cologne, Germany; Laboratory for Developmental and Regenerative RNA Biology, Center for Molecular Medicine (CMMC), University of Cologne, Cologne, Germany*

ALBRECHT BINDEREIF • *Institute of Biochemistry, Department of Biology and Chemistry, Justus Liebig University Giessen, Giessen, Germany*

JES-NIELS BOECKEL • *Institute for Cardiomyopathies, Division of Cardiology, Department of Internal Medicine III, University Clinic Heidelberg, Heidelberg, Germany*

ANASTASIYA BOLTENGAGEN • *Systems Biology of Gene-Regulatory Elements, Berlin Institute for Medical Systems Biology (BIMSB), Max Delbrück Center (MDC) for Molecular Medicine in the Helmholtz Association, Berlin, Germany*

BING CHEN • *Fudan University Shanghai Cancer Center, Institutes of Biomedical Sciences and Shanghai Medical College, Fudan University, Shanghai, China*

SIMON J. CONN • *Centre for Cancer Biology, An Alliance Between University of South Australia and SA Health, Adelaide, SA, Australia*

VANESSA CONN • *Centre for Cancer Biology, An Alliance Between University of South Australia and SA Health, Adelaide, SA, Australia*

DAPHNE A. COOPER • *Department of Biology, University of Nevada, Reno, Reno, NV, USA*

MARIELA CORTÉS-LÓPEZ • *Department of Biology, University of Nevada, Reno, Reno, NV, USA*

CHRISTOPH DIETERICH • *Section of Bioinformatics and Systems Cardiology, Department of Internal Medicine III, Klaus Tschira Institute for Integrative Computational Cardiology, University Hospital Heidelberg, Heidelberg, Germany; German Center for Cardiovascular Research (DZHK)—Partner site Heidelberg/Mannheim, Heidelberg, Germany*

DAWOOD B. DUDEKULA • *Laboratory of Genetics and Genomics, National Institute on Aging-Intramural Research Program, National Institutes of Health, Baltimore, MD, USA*

GREGORY J. GOODALL • *Centre for Cancer Biology, An Alliance Between University of South Australia and SA Health, Adelaide, SA, Australia*

MYRIAM GOROSPE • *Laboratory of Genetics and Genomics, National Institute on Aging-Intramural Research Program, National Institutes of Health, Baltimore, MD, USA*

THOMAS B. HANSEN • *Department of Molecular Biology and Genetics (MBG), Interdisciplinary Nanoscience Center (iNANO), Aarhus University, Aarhus, Denmark*

ANDREAS W. HEUMÜLLER • *Institute for Cardiovascular Regeneration, University Frankfurt, Frankfurt, Germany*

SHENLING HUANG • *Fudan University Shanghai Cancer Center, Institutes of Biomedical Sciences and Shanghai Medical College, Fudan University, Shanghai, China*

TOBIAS JAKOBI • *Section of Bioinformatics and Systems Cardiology, Department of Internal Medicine III, Klaus Tschira Institute for Integrative Computational Cardiology, University Hospital Heidelberg, Heidelberg, Germany; German Center for Cardiovascular Research (DZHK)—Partner site Heidelberg/Mannheim, Heidelberg, Germany*

CHRISTINE KOCKS • *Systems Biology of Gene-Regulatory Elements, Berlin Institute for Medical Systems Biology (BIMSB), Max Delbrück Center (MDC) for Molecular Medicine in the Helmholtz Association, Berlin, Germany*

AYUMI KODAMA • *Department of Chemistry, Graduate School of Science, Nagoya University, Nagoya, Japan*

LEO KURIAN • *Cologne Excellence Cluster on Cellular Stress Responses in Aging-Associated Diseases, University of Cologne, Cologne, Germany; Institute for Neurophysiology, University of Cologne, Cologne, Germany; Laboratory for Developmental and Regenerative RNA Biology, Center for Molecular Medicine (CMMC), University of Cologne, Cologne, Germany*

YAN LI • *Fudan University Shanghai Cancer Center, Institutes of Biomedical Sciences, Shanghai Medical College, Fudan University, Shanghai, China*

DAWEI LIU • *Centre for Cancer Biology, An Alliance Between University of South Australia and SA Health, Adelaide, SA, Australia*

PEDRO MIURA • *Department of Biology, University of Nevada, Reno, Reno, NV, USA*

SABINE MÜLLER • *Institut für Biochemie, Universität Greifswald, Greifswald, Germany*

AMARESH C. PANDA • *Laboratory of Genetics and Genomics, National Institute on Aging-Intramural Research Program, National Institutes of Health, Baltimore, MD, USA*

ARGYRIS PAPANTONIS • *Chromatin Systems Biology Laboratory, Center for Molecular Medicine Cologne (CMMC), University of Cologne, Cologne, Germany*

SONJA PETKOVIC • *Institut für Molekulare Medizin, UK S-H, Campus Lübeck, Universität zu Lübeck, Lübeck, Germany*

MONIKA PIEWECKA • *Systems Biology of Gene-Regulatory Elements, Berlin Institute for Medical Systems Biology (BIMSB), Max Delbrück Center (MDC) for Molecular Medicine in the Helmholtz Association, Berlin, Germany*

CHRISTIAN PREUSSER • *Institute of Biochemistry, Department of Biology and Chemistry, Justus Liebig University Giessen, Giessen, Germany*

NIKOLAUS RAJEWSKY • *Systems Biology of Gene-Regulatory Elements, Berlin Institute for Medical Systems Biology (BIMSB), Max Delbrück Center (MDC) for Molecular Medicine in the Helmholtz Association, Berlin, Germany*

OLIVER ROSSBACH • *Institute of Biochemistry, Department of Biology and Chemistry, Justus Liebig University Giessen, Giessen, Germany*

AGNIESZKA RYBAK-WOLF • *Systems Biology of Gene-Regulatory Elements, Berlin Institute for Medical Systems Biology (BIMSB), Max Delbrück Center (MDC) for Molecular Medicine in the Helmholtz Association, Berlin, Germany*

TIM SCHNEIDER • *Institute of Biochemistry, Department of Biology and Chemistry, Justus Liebig University Giessen, Giessen, Germany*

SILKE SCHREINER • *Institute of Biochemistry, Department of Biology and Chemistry, Justus Liebig University Giessen, Giessen, Germany*

GE SHAN • *The CAS Key Laboratory of Innate Immunity and Chronic Disease, CAS Center for Excellence in Molecular Cell Science, School of Life Sciences, University of Science and Technology of China, Hefei, Anhui Province, China*

XIAOLIN WANG • *The CAS Key Laboratory of Innate Immunity and Chronic Disease, CAS Center for Excellence in Molecular Cell Science, School of Life Sciences, University of Science and Technology of China, Hefei, Anhui Province, China*

ZEFENG WANG • *CAS Key Lab for Computational Biology, CAS-MPG Partner Institute for Computational Biology, Shanghai, China; CAS Center for Excellence in Molecular Cell Science, Shanghai Institute for Biological Sciences, Chinese Academy of Sciences, Shanghai, China*

JIAN-HUA YANG • *Key Laboratory of Gene Engineering of the Ministry of Education, Guangzhou, People's Republic of China; State Key Laboratory for Biocontrol, Sun Yat-sen University, Guangzhou, People's Republic of China*

YUN YANG • *CAS Key Lab for Computational Biology, CAS-MPG Partner Institute for Computational Biology, Shanghai, China*

XIAO-QIN ZHANG • *School of Medicine, South China University of Technology, Guangzhou, People's Republic of China; Department of Surgery, Li Ka Shing Faculty of Medicine, University of Hong Kong, Pok Fu Lam, Hong Kong*

FANGQING ZHAO • *Computational Genomics Lab, Beijing Institutes of Life Science, Chinese Academy of Sciences, Beijing, China*

YI ZHENG • *Computational Genomics Lab, Beijing Institutes of Life Science, Chinese Academy of Sciences, Beijing, China*

ANNE ZIRKEL • *Laboratory for Systems Biology of Chromatin, Center for Molecular Medicine Cologne (CMMC), University of Cologne, Cologne, Germany*

Chapter 1

Detection and Reconstruction of Circular RNAs from Transcriptomic Data

Yi Zheng and Fangqing Zhao

Abstract

Recent studies have shown that circular RNAs (circRNAs) are a novel class of abundant, stable, and ubiquitous noncoding RNA molecules in eukaryotic organisms. Comprehensive detection and reconstruction of circRNAs from high-throughput transcriptome data is an initial step to study their biogenesis and function. Several tools have been developed to deal with this issue, but they require many steps and are difficult to use. To solve this problem, we provide a protocol for researchers to detect and reconstruct circRNA by employing CIRI2, CIRI-AS, and CIRI-full. This protocol can not only simplify the usage of above tools but also integrate their results.

Key words Circular RNA (circRNA), Transcript reconstruction

1 Introduction

Over the past few years, high-throughput RNA-seq data analysis and corresponding experimental validation have proved that circular RNAs (circRNAs) are ubiquitous in eukaryotic organisms and some of them undertake essential biological functions instead of transcriptional noises [1–5]. For example, CDR1as can function as microRNA sponges [2, 4]. circEIF3J and circPPAIP2 can enhance the expression of their parental genes [6]. cir-ITCH plays a role in colorectal cancer by regulating the Wnt/β-catenin pathway [7]. However, the structure and function of the majority of circRNAs are still unknown. To further explore the diversity and function of circRNAs, an all-around computational tool is urgently required to dig out these cryptic molecules from high-throughput but fragmented transcriptomic data.

Currently existing circRNA detection methods are all based on identification of back-spliced junction (BSJ) reads, and they can be divided into annotation-dependent (such as MapSplice, CIRCexplorer, and KNIFE) and de novo (such as find-circ, segemehl, and CIRI) algorithms [4, 8–12]. These methods are

Christoph Dieterich and Argyris Papantonis (eds.), *Circular RNAs: Methods and Protocols*, Methods in Molecular Biology, vol. 1724, https://doi.org/10.1007/978-1-4939-7562-4_1, © Springer Science+Business Media, LLC 2018

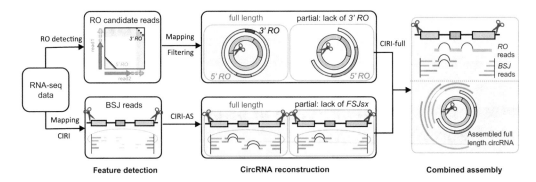

Fig. 1 The workflow of the CIRI pipeline. RO reads and BSJ reads are firstly detected from RNA-seq data. Full length of circRNAs can be reconstructed when both 5′ and 3′ RO are present or they are completely covered by BSJ reads. For those lacking 3′RO or FSJs, a combined assembly will be performed to integrate both 5′ RO reads and BSJ reads

used not only for a direct investigation of circRNA loci but also as basis of more complicated analyses. For example, our previous method CIRI facilitated the development of another algorithm (CIRI-AS) on characterizing internal structure and alternative splicing within circRNAs by providing BSJs and corresponding reads [13]. Most recently, we have developed a new tool, CIRI-full, for effective reconstruction of full-length circRNAs from the transcriptome. Through extensive evaluations of simulated, real transcriptomic datasets, we demonstrated that CIRI-full exhibits excellent performance in circRNA identification and whole-sequence reconstruction. In addition, the updated version of CIRI employed an adapted maximum likelihood estimation based on multiple seed matching to identify back-spliced junction reads and to filter false positives derived from repetitive sequences and mapping errors. Through objective assessment criteria based on real data from RNase R-treated samples, it was demonstrated that CIRI2 outperformed its previous version CIRI and all other widely used tools, featured with remarkably balanced sensitivity, reliability, duration, and RAM usage [14].

In this chapter, we provide a protocol for detecting and reconstructing circRNAs from RNA-seq data using the CIRI pipeline, which combines three tools, CIRI2, CIRI-AS, and CIRI-full (Fig. 1). This protocol will help users simplify the process of circRNA detection and reconstruction.

2   Materials

2.1   Hardware and Environment

To run the CIRI pipeline, a server or PC with Linux or Mac OS X operation system is required. For a large RNase R-treated dataset (e.g., SRR444975 with 41 Gb sequences), at least 10 GB RAM is required. When using multi-threading, more RAM will be needed [14]. Additionally, Perl (version ≥ 5.8) and Java (version > 1.6) should be installed to execute some of the software in this protocol.

2.2 Tool Requirements

Four tools are used in the CIRI pipeline: CIRI2 (https://sourceforge.net/projects/ciri/), a chiastic clipping signal-based algorithm, which can detect circRNAs from transcriptome data by employing multiple filtration strategies [14]; CIRI_AS (https://sourceforge.net/projects/ciri/), a detection tool for circRNA internal components and alternative splicing events [13]; CIRI-full (https://sourceforge.net/projects/ciri-full/), a new tool to reconstruct full-length circRNAs from RNA-seq datasets; BWA (https://sourceforge.net/projects/bio-bwa/files/), a read mapping tool, which generates SAM file of split mapping results for the CIRI pipeline.

The latest versions of CIRI2 and CIRI-AS have been already packed with the CIRI-full package. BWA should be installed following the instruction of its manual and then should be added to $path.

2.3 Data Requirements

The input files for the CIRI pipeline include RNA-seq data, reference genome, and reference genome annotation. RNA-seq data should be generated using the RiboMinus RNA samples with or without RNase R treatment. However, when using poly(A)-enriched RNA-seq datasets, the CIRI pipeline may detect only very few circRNAs. If the datasets are downloaded from public database (e.g., SRA), here is an example showing how to preprocess the public RNA-seq data archived in SRA. First, download the SRA Toolkit that is suitable to your system from the following address (https://www.ncbi.nlm.nih.gov/sra/docs/toolkitsoft/) and then enter the dictionary:

    cd sratoolkit.2.8.1-3-mac64/

Type the following command to download the SRA file by using prefetch in the SRA Toolkit.

    bin/prefetch SRR1636985

The SRA file will be saved at this dictionary: ~/ncbi/public/sra/
Then, covert the SRA file into FASTQ format by using fastq-dump using the following command:

    bin/fastq-dump --split-files ~/ncbi/public/sra/SRR1636985.sra

Two files, SRR1636985_1.fastq and SRR1636985_2.fastq, will be generated in the current directory. These two files can be imported to the CIRI pipeline for identifying circRNAs.
Please note that the reads of a pair of FASTQ files should be in equal length. If the reads are in low quality, all of the reads in these FASTQ files should be trimmed into the same length. Before

running the CIRI pipeline, removing rRNA reads will significantly reduce the time usage of CIRI.

To filter false-positive BSJ reads, the CIRI pipeline will load reference sequences to check whether AG and GT dinucleotides (or reverse complementary dinucleotides CT and AC) flank segments of a junction on the reference genome. Considering splicing signals for minor introns such as AT-AC and other possible situations where GT-AG splicing signals are not applicable, the CIRI pipeline can extract exon boundary positions from a GTF annotation file provided by users and use them as a complementary or an alternative filter for false positives. Candidate junction reads not supported by splicing signals or exon boundaries are filtered out. Reference genome sequence in the FASTA format (in a single file) and reference annotation file in the GTF format can be downloaded from the ENSEMBL website (www.ensembl. org) or Gencode website (http://www.gencodegenes.org). It should be noted that the sequence file and its annotation file should be in the same version. For example, if the GRCh37 genome sequence was downloaded at ftp://ftp.ensembl.org/pub/release-75//fasta/homo_sapiens/dna/Homo_sapiens.GRCh37.75.dna.primary_assembly.fa.gz, its annotation GTF file should be downloaded from the same folder as well (ftp://ftp.ensembl.org/pub/release-75//gtf/homo_sapiens/Homo_sapiens.GRCh37.75.gtf.gz).

3   Method: How to Run the CIRI Pipeline

3.1   Running the CIRI Pipeline Step by Step on the Test Dataset

Step 1: Enter the directory where you download CIRI-full and type the following command in your terminal to unzip the package:

unzip CIRI-full.zip

cd CIRI-full

Step 2: Make index for BWA mem using the following command. In this protocol, the test data archived in the CIRI-full package is used as an example. If the reference genome is large, please add the option "-a bwtsw".

bwa index test_ref.fa

Then, align reads to the reference genome using bwa mem. An example command is shown as below:

bwa mem -T 19 test_ref.fa test_1.fq.gz test_2.fq.gz > test_output/test.sam

Users can add "-t number" option to run BWA mem with multiple threads, which will greatly reduce the running time of BWA.

Step 3: Running CIRI to detect circRNAs from the SAM alignment. The recommended usage of CIRI is shown as below:

```
perl ../bin/CIRI_v2.0.4.pl -I test_output/test.sam -O test_output/test.ciri -F test_ref.fa -A test_anno.gtf
```

If the hardware has multiple CPUs and sufficient RAM resources, users can use multiple threads by adding "-T number". To detect very-low-abundance circRNAs, setting option "-0" will output all circRNAs regardless junction read counts or PCC signals. For more options, please use "-help" or "-H" options or check CIRI's manual.

Step 4: Running CIRI-AS to identify the cirexons in circRNAs by analyzing the mapping position of BSJ reads. "test.ciri" file is generated by CIRI, which contains all identified circRNAs. Recommended command of CIRI-AS is shown as below:

```
perl ../bin/CIRI_AS_v1.2.pl -S test_output/test.sam -C test_output/test.ciri -F test_ref.fa -A test_anno.gtf -O test_output/test -D yes
```

Compared with CIRI, CIRI-AS requires much less CPU resource and always finish in dozens of minutes. It will output a detailed list of mapping positions of BSJ reads, coverage, as well as the cirexons in circRNAs when using "–D yes" option.

Step 5: Running CIRI-full to reconstruct full-length circRNAs. CIRI-full firstly detects Reverse Overlap (RO) reads from inputted RNA-seq read pairs. Then, these candidate RO reads will be merged into long reads. The command of this step is shown as follows:

```
java -jar ../CIRI-full.jar RO1 -1 test_1.fq.gz -2 test_2.fq.gz -o test_output/test
```

The threshold of detecting RO feature can be adjusted by using options "-minM" and "-minI", which represents the minimal match length of RO region and minimal identity% of RO region, respectively. The output file which contains candidate long reads will be named with "_ro1.fq" suffix.

Step 6: Using BWA mem to map the RO candidate long reads to the reference genome. The command is shown as below:

```
bwa mem -T 19 test_ref.fa test_output/test_ro1.fq > test_output/test_ro1.sam
```

Step 7: Running CIRI-full's RO2 module to analyze the mapping information of candidate long reads. After filtering, CIRI-full algorithms will output the reads that can cover full length of circRNAs, and the location of every component inside circRNAs. The command of this step is shown as below:

java -jar ../CIRI-full.jar RO2 -r test_ref.fa -s test_output/test_ro1.sam -l 250 -o test_output/test

"-l 250" option represents the sequencing length of inputted RNA-seq reads. The output file is named with "-ro2_info.list" suffix, which shows a detailed list of RO reads and their locations on the reference genome.

Step 8: Merging the results of CIRI-AS and CIRI-full. Considering that CIRI-AS and CIRI-full use different features to identify circRNAs, they can complement each other by detecting different kinds of circRNAs. Therefore, in this step, CIRI-full will perform a combined assembly by merging all circRNAs detected using the two methods. Here is the command:

java -jar ../CIRI-full.jar Merge -c test_output/test.ciri -as test_output/test_jav.list -ro test_output/test_ro2_info.list -a test_anno.gtf -r test_ref.fa -o test_output/test

3.2 An Automated Pipeline for Detecting and Reconstructing circRNAs

To simplify above procedures, we develop an automated pipeline to run all commands in a batch mode. Considering that in this pipeline CIRI2 and CIRI-full will be run at the same time, more RAM and CPU resources are required. The procedures are shown as follows:

Step 1: Enter the directory where you download CIRI-full and type the following command in your terminal to unzip the package:

unzip CIRI-full.zip
cd CIRI-full

Step 2: Index the reference genome using BWA.

cd CIRI-full_test
bwa index test_ref.fa

Step 3: To run the automated CIRI pipeline, please type the following command:

java -jar ../CIRI-full.jar Pipeline -1 test_1.fq.gz -2 test_2.fq.gz -a test_anno.gtf -r test_ref.fa -d test_output/ -o test

Details of all available options are included in the manual of CIRI-full, or type the following command to check the usage of this algorithm:

java –jar CIRI-full.jar Pipeline -h

Other options can be adjusted according to user's requirement: -0 (output all circRNAs including those with only one BSJ read support), -t number (number of threads used in CIRI and BWA mem).

3.3 Output of the CIRI-Full Pipeline

If you are using the automated pipeline, the output files will be put under the directory set by "-d" option. Four folders will be created under this directory: "CIRI_output/", "CIRI-AS_output/", "CIRI-full_output/", and "sam/", which contains the output files of CIRI, CIRI-AS, CIRI-full, and bwa. The two final files are in the "CIRI-full_ouput/" folder, which are:

prefix_merge_circRNA.anno

prefix_merge_full_circRNA.fa

"prefix" can be set by "-o" option.

"prefix_merge_circRNA.anno" contains the reconstructed state of circRNAs. The cirexons of fully reconstructed circRNA are shown. For partially reconstructed circRNA, predicted cirexons and estimated length are also presented. Columns are separated by tabs:

#CircRNA_ID #BSJ #Start #End #Expression #Gene #GTF-annotated_Exon #Cirexon #If_reconstructed #Length #Predicted_length #IF Constructed_by_BSJ/RO_reads

In #Predict_length column, the length of partially reconstructed circRNAs is calculated by summing the length of reconstructed cirexons and the estimated length of unreconstructed cirexons. In #If_reconstructed column, "Full" indicates that entire sequence of a circRNA is reconstructed. "Almost" indicates that more than 70% of the sequence of a circRNA is reconstructed. "Part" means that less than 70% of the sequence of a circRNA is reconstructed.

"prefix_merge_full_circRNA.fa" contains the FASTA-formatted sequence of reconstructed full-length circRNAs.

Some intermediate files also provide useful information. The output file "prefix.ciri" generated by CIRI contains a list of circRNAs with their location, expression level, and annotation. The output file "prefix.list" generated by CIRI-AS shows all predicted cirexons for each circRNA. "prefix_AS.list" shows alternatively spliced events and the PSI values of circRNAs. "prefix_jav.list" (using option –D yes) contains the mapping locations of all BSJ reads. The file "prefix_ro2_info.list" shows the mapping information of RO reads. For detailed information of these files, users can refer to the manuals of CIRI2, CIRI-AS, and CIRI-full.

Acknowledgments

This work was supported by NSFC grants (91640117, 91531306) and CAS grants to FZ.

Reference

1. Ashwal-Fluss R, Meyer M, Pamudurti NR, Ivanov A, Bartok O, Hanan M, Evantal N, Memczak S, Rajewsky N, Kadener S (2014) circRNA biogenesis competes with pre-mRNA splicing. Mol Cell 56:55–66

2. Hansen TB, Jensen TI, Clausen BH, Bramsen JB, Finsen B, Damgaard CK, Kjems J (2013) Natural RNA circles function as efficient microRNA sponges. Nature 495:384–388

3. Jeck WR, Sorrentino JA, Wang K, Slevin MK, Burd CE, Liu J, Marzluff WF, Sharpless NE (2013) Circular RNAs are abundant, conserved, and associated with ALU repeats. RNA 19:141–157

4. Memczak S, Jens M, Elefsinioti A, Torti F, Krueger J, Rybak A, Maier L, Mackowiak SD, Gregersen LH, Munschauer M et al (2013) Circular RNAs are a large class of animal RNAs with regulatory potency. Nature 495:333–338

5. Salzman J, Gawad C, Wang PL, Lacayo N, Brown PO (2012) Circular RNAs are the predominant transcript isoform from hundreds of human genes in diverse cell types. PLoS One 7:e30733

6. Li Z, Huang C, Bao C, Chen L, Lin M, Wang X, Zhong G, Yu B, Hu W, Dai L et al (2015) Exon-intron circular RNAs regulate transcription in the nucleus. Nat Struct Mol Biol 22:256–264

7. Li F, Zhang L, Li W, Deng J, Zheng J, An M, Lu J, Zhou Y (2015) Circular RNA ITCH has inhibitory effect on ESCC by suppressing the Wnt/beta-catenin pathway. Oncotarget 6:6001–6013

8. Hoffmann S, Otto C, Kurtz S, Sharma CM, Khaitovich P, Vogel J, Stadler PF, Hackermuller J (2009) Fast mapping of short sequences with mismatches, insertions and deletions using index structures. PLoS Comput Biol 5:e1000502

9. Gao Y, Wang J, Zhao F (2015) CIRI: an efficient and unbiased algorithm for de novo circular RNA identification. Genome Biol 16:4

10. Hoffmann S, Otto C, Doose G, Tanzer A, Langenberger D, Christ S, Kunz M, Holdt LM, Teupser D, Hackermuller J, Stadler PF (2014) A multi-split mapping algorithm for circular RNA, splicing, trans-splicing and fusion detection. Genome Biol 15:R34

11. Zhang XO, Wang HB, Zhang Y, Lu X, Chen LL, Yang L (2014) Complementary sequence-mediated exon circularization. Cell 159:134–147

12. Szabo L, Morey R, Palpant NJ, Wang PL, Afari N, Jiang C, Parast MM, Murry CE, Laurent LC, Salzman J (2015) Statistically based splicing detection reveals neural enrichment and tissue-specific induction of circular RNA during human fetal development. Genome Biol 16:126

13. Gao Y, Wang J, Zheng Y, Zhang J, Chen S, Zhao F (2016) Comprehensive identification of internal structure and alternative splicing events in circular RNAs. Nat Commun 7:12060

14. Gao Y, Zhang J, Zhao F (2017) Circular RNA identification based on multiple seed matching. Brief Bioinform. https://doi.org/10.1093/bib/bbx014

Chapter 2

Deep Computational Circular RNA Analytics from RNA-seq Data

Tobias Jakobi and Christoph Dieterich

Abstract

Circular RNAs (circRNAs) have been first described as "scrambled exons" in the 1990s. CircRNAs originate from back splicing or exon skipping of linear RNA templates and have continuously gained attention in recent years due to the availability of high-throughput whole-transcriptome sequencing methods. Numerous manuscripts describe thousands of circRNAs throughout uni- and multicellular eukaryote species and demonstrated that they are conserved, stable, and abundant in specific tissues or conditions. This manuscript provides a walk-through of our bioinformatics toolbox, which covers all aspects of in silico circRNA analysis, starting from raw sequencing data and back-splicing junction discovery to circRNA quantitation and reconstruction of internal the circRNA structure.

Key words Bioinformatics, Whole-transcriptome sequencing, Circular RNA detection, Circular, RNA analysis

1 Introduction

Compared to other branches of bioinformatics, in silico circRNA analysis still is a young field. First tools to detect circRNAs from sequencing data were published in the early 2010s; however most of the currently employed tools are of newer origin [1–4, 6–10]. Common to basically all detection algorithms is the requirement for one or more external programs that are providing read mapping functions. Common choices for read mapping tools are STAR [11], bowtie2 [12], and bwa [13]. All three mapping tools are suitable for paired-end sequencing, while STAR is also splice-site aware, meaning that the program is able correctly to align reads or read pairs that cover splice junctions, a feature especially important for work with circRNAs.

Back-splicing junctions can be detected from rRNA-depleted whole-transcriptome sequencing data. CircRNAs typically do not contain a poly-A tail and are resistant to exonuclease treatment. Jeck and Sharpless proposed a circRNA optimized sequencing

Christoph Dieterich and Argyris Papantonis (eds.), *Circular RNAs: Methods and Protocols*, Methods in Molecular Biology, vol. 1724, https://doi.org/10.1007/978-1-4939-7562-4_2, © Springer Science+Business Media, LLC 2018

protocol termed "CircleSeq" that was quickly established as gold standard [14]. CircleSeq exploits the fact that circRNAs are resistant to degradation by the RNase R enzyme. The rRNA-depleted RNA sample is divided into treated and mock-treated sample: RNA within the treated sample is digested whereas the untreated sample only receives a mock treatment with water. Both samples are subsequently sequenced and compared. Given this setup, it is expected that the sequenced mock-treated sample contains reads originating from the complete RNA pool, including linear RNAs, while the treated sample's reads should be enriched for circRNAs due to the RNase R-based depletion of linear RNA fragments.

We present a general work, starting with a stringent quality control of the obtained sequencing data. It is crucial to assess the data quality as later steps of the analysis pipeline may otherwise fail or, even worse, silently produce flawed data. The quality control is usually followed by the alignment step that provides BAM files consisting of compressed and aligned reads required for deep inspection in follow-up steps. The work flow described within this manuscript employs the DCC/CircTest software for circRNA detection and enrichment testing [9] combined with FUCHS [15] to reconstruct the complete exon/intron structure of circRNAs.

2   Materials

2.1   Required Hardware and Environment

In order to perform read alignments on human genome scale with STAR an ×86–64-based machine with a 64bit Linux/Mac OS operating system and at least 30GB of RAM is required. The read mapping step depicts the bottleneck of the work flow requiring most resources; thus all subsequent steps will also perform well on the specified hardware. The work flow shown in this work was performed on a Debian Linux 8.6 (jessie) system but should run on any other Linux distribution without further problems.

2.2   Required Software Environment

The following software is required to run all parts of the work flow: STAR, R, and Python are normally available as prepackaged binary download and need not to be compiled from source. Our Python-based tools DCC and FUCHS are installed from source code but the compilation procedure is carried out by an automatic installer.

- The STAR read aligner, obtainable directly from GitHub via https://github.com/alexdobin/STAR
- The Bowtie2 read aligner, hosted on Sourceforge: https://sourceforge.net/projects/bowtie-bio/files/bowtie2/2.3.0/
- SAMtools [16], the universal SAM/BAM file manipulation tools, obtainable via http://www.htslib.org/download/

- The R environment for statistical computing [17], either via package manager of the employed Linux distribution or directly via https://cran.r-project.org/bin/linux/

- A working Python (2.7) environment, including the pip installer either via package manager of the employed Linux distribution or directly via https://www.python.org/downloads/release/python-2712/

- DCC circRNA detection tool, obtainable via GitHub: https://github.com/dieterich-lab/DCC

- FUCHS, a circRNA reconstruction tool, obtainable via https://github.com/dieterich-lab/FUCHS

- CircTest, a circRNA testing and plotting R package, obtainable via https://github.com/dieterich-lab/CircTest

- FastQC [18], a quality control tool for sequencing reads, obtainable via http://www.bioinformatics.babraham.ac.uk/projects/download.html#fastqc

- FlexBar [5], a trimming tool allowing to remove residual adapter sequences from sequencing reads, obtainable via https://github.com/seqan/flexbar

- [Optional] CircleSeq raw data used in this example work flow for RNaseR enrichment testing from murine heart tissue [19], via the NCBI SRA, https://www.ncbi.nlm.nih.gov/sra/, accession SRP071584

- [Optional] Long RNA-Seq raw data used in this example work flow for full circle reconstruction, via the NCBI SRA, https://www.ncbi.nlm.nih.gov/sra/, accession SRP097141

3   Methods

3.1   Quality Control of Obtained Sequencing Data with FastQC

The tool FastQC is designed to carry out routine checks of sequencing data, including crucial information like GC content, read length distribution, remaining adapter sequences, or overrepresented sequences. A typical call for FastQC to analyze all sequencing files in the current directory could be

```
> cd /path/to/sequencing/files/
> fastqc *.fastq.gz -t 4
```

In the above call to FastQC it is assumed that all raw data files are gzipped FASTQ files (hence *.fastq.gz) and up to 4 processors on the system are employed for the analysis (-t 4). Although warnings generated by FastQC are relatively conservative, user should pay attention to the details and make sure that the data does not include any obvious problems like below-average read quality and/or very high sequence duplication levels.

3.2 Residual Adapter Removal with FlexBar

FlexBar is designed to remove parts of the sequencing adapter remaining in the reads after sequencing. These residual sequence parts are interfering with the read mapping process and may significantly reduce the mapping rate, i.e., the percentage of reads aligning to the reference genome. It is important to keep in mind the sequencing library setup from this step on since the commands used for paired-end datasets differ from the single-end data processing steps. In the following example FlexBar call a paired-end library is assumed:

```
flexbar -r mate_1.fastq.gz -p mate_2.fastq.gz -t / path/
to/output/folder/filename.fastq -n 20 -z GZ -m 30 -u 0 -q
TAIL -qt 28 -a AGATCGGAAGAG -qf sanger
```

The above command would run FlexBar on 20 processors (−n 20), providing both mates of the sequencing run via -r (mate 1) and -p (mate 2) using a generic Illumina adapter sequence (−a AGATCGGAAGAG), latest Illumina quality scores (−qf sanger), and a very conservative minimal quality score of 28 (−qt 28). This step has to be carried out for all samples in the library.

3.3 Removal of Remaining Ribosomal RNA from Sequencing Data

Even if the input RNA has been treated with ribosomal RNA removal kits prior to sequencing, our experience shows that treated samples still tend to contain considerable amounts of reads mapping to ribosomal RNA. Ribosomal RNA is highly abundant and may confound overall analysis results. We employ bowtie2 to map all adapter-free reads against an artificial reference solely consisting of rRNA sequences. Only reads not mapping against this rRNA reference are part of follow-up analysis steps. A first step is the generation of the index bowtie2 uses for read alignment:

```
# download sample fasta file containing mus musculus
ribosomal RNA sequences (GI: 511668571):
> wget https://github.com/dieterich-lab/circular-rna-
book/blob/master/data/mmusculus.rRNA.fasta
# generate an rRNA index for bowtie2
> bowtie2-build mmusculus.rRNA.fasta mmusculus.rRNA
```

In a second step, the generated index can now be used to filter out rRNA reads and write the remaining reads in separate files:

```
# align reads against the rRNA reference in paired
end fashion
> bowtie2 -x mmusculus.rRNA -1 mate_1.fastq.1 -2
mate_2.fastq.2 -no-unal --threads 20 --un-conc-gz /
path/to/output/directory/adapter_removed_rRNA_
filtered.fastq.gz
```

In this example, bowtie2 uses the index just created (-x mmusculus.rRNA) while input read files processed by FlexBar are supplied via −1 mate_1.fastq.1 −2 mate_2.fastq.2.

The tool will employ 20 processors (—threads 20) and write non-aligned reads (i.e., the rRNA-free reads) into the file supplied via `--un-conc-gz /path/to/output/directory/adapter_removed_ rRNA_filtered.fastq.gz`

3.4 Principal Read Mapping with STAR

Mapping reads to the destination reference genome is the most resource-intensive part of the work flow and as such reasonable hardware is recommended. Similar to the bowtie2 step an index needs to be created. In contrast to the very small index constructed to remove rRNA mapping reads however, the STAR index has to include the whole reference genome. The index only needs to be created once which puts the relatively long construction time into perspective. Since the sequencing reads we employ for this example originate from *Mus musculus* the reference genome has to be obtained:

```
# download the reference genome fasta file from the
ENSEMBL FTP

> wget ftp://ftp.ensembl.org/pub/current_fasta/mus_
musculus/dna/Mus_musculus.GRCm38.dna.toplevel.fa.gz

# download the reference genome annotation file from
the ENSEMBL FTP

> wget ftp://ftp.ensembl.org/pub/current_gtf/mus_
musculus/Mus_musculus.GRCm38.87.gtf.gz

# decompress gzipped fasta file and gzipped annota-
tion file

gzip -d Mus_musculus.GRCm38.dna.fa.gz

gzip -d Mus_musculus.GRCm38.87.gtf.gz

# create the STAR index [may take some time]

STAR --runThreadN 20 --runMode genomeGener-
ate --genomeDir /path/to/genome/index/ --genomeFas-
taFiles

Mus_musculus.GRCm38.dna.fa
```

Here, STAR is run on 20 CPUs for the index creation (`--run-ThreadN 20`), the input reference genome is specified via `--genome-FastaFiles`, and an output directory is specified using the `--genomeDir` parameter.

Again, as for bowtie2 the read pairs (or single reads) need to be aligned against the reference genome. Inputs for the STAR alignment step are adapter-trimmed and rRNA-free reads from the first two steps. In order to align paired-end reads the following STAR command should be used:

```
> STAR --runThreadN 20 \
        --genomeDir /path/to/genome/index/ \
        --outSAMtype BAM SortedByCoordinate \
        --readFilesIn mate_1.fastq.gz mate_2.fastq.gz \
```

```
        --readFilesCommand zcat \
        --outFileNamePrefix /path/to/star/output/ \
        --outReadsUnmapped Fastx \
        --outSJfilterOverhangMin 15 15 15 15 \
        --alignSJoverhangMin 15 \
        --sjdbGTFfile Mus_musculus.GRCm38.87.gtf \
        --alignSJDBoverhangMin 15 \
        --outFilterMultimapNmax 20 \
        --outFilterScoreMin 1 \
        --outFilterMatchNmin 1 \
        --outFilterMismatchNmax 2 \
        --chimSegmentMin 15 \
        --chimScoreMin 15 \
        --chimScoreSeparation 10 \
        --chimJunctionOverhangMin 15 \
```

As for the index creation, 20 CPUs are employed to speed up the mapping process. STAR significantly profits from multiprocessing, as also bowtie2 does. The `--readFilesIn` parameter takes two file arguments, mate 1 and mate 2 reads separated by a space. The annotation is provided via `--sjdbGTFfile Mus_musculus.GRCm38.87.gtf`, allowing STAR to honor splice junctions correctly. Since the input read files are gzipped furthermore `--readFilesCommand zcat` is specified. In order to be able to harmonize optimally with the DCC circRNA detection, STAR is instructed to save results directly as sorted, compressed BAM file (`--outSAMtype BAM SortedByCoordinate`). Other parameters seen in the listing above are optimized for usage with the DCC software and should only be changed by advanced users. DCC recommends that paired-end datasets are mapped three times, (1) using both mates together, (2) using only mate 1, and (3) using only mate 2. In order to map only the first mate (mate 1) the following code can be used:

```
> STAR --runThreadN 20 \
        --genomeDir /path/to/genome/index/ \
        --outSAMtype BAM SortedByCoordinate \
        --readFilesIn mate_1.fastq.gz \
        --readFilesCommand zcat \
        --outFileNamePrefix /path/to/star/output/ \
        --outReadsUnmapped Fastx \
        --outSJfilterOverhangMin 15 15 15 15 \
        --alignSJoverhangMin 15 \
        --sjdbGTFfile Mus_musculus.GRCm38.87.gtf \
        --alignSJDBoverhangMin 15 \
```

```
--outFilterMultimapNmax 20 \
--outFilterScoreMin 1 \
--outFilterMatchNmin 1 \
--outFilterMismatchNmax 2 \
--chimSegmentMin 15 \
--chimScoreMin 15 \
--chimScoreSeparation 10 \
--chimJunctionOverhangMin 15 \
```

The command for mate 2 is identical with the exception of providing the second mate read file (mate 2). After this step, three different STAR output directories should exist for each sample of the library.

3.5 CircRNA Detection with DCC

DCC is a python package intended to detect and quantify circRNAs with high specificity. DCC works with the STAR's `chimeric.out.junction` files which contain chimerical aligned reads including circRNA back-splice junction spanning reads. DCC depends on `pysam`, `pandas`, `numpy`, and `HTSeq`. The installation process of DCC will automatically check for the dependencies and install or update missing (Python) packages. The following command will install DCC for the currently logged-in user:

```
> git clone https://github.com/dieterich-lab/DCC.git
> cd DCC Principal read mapping with STAR
> python setup.py install --user
# test if the installation was successful
> DCC --version
0.4.4
```

Before circRNA detection with DCC can be performed, several input files have to be prepared in order for DCC to work correctly:

1. A so-called `samplesheet` file, containing either the absolute or the relative paths to the `chimeric.out.junction` produced by STAR for the paired-end run of each library [Command line flag: `@samplesheet`]

2. A GTF-formatted annotation of repetitive regions which is used to filter out circRNA candidates from repetitive regions. [Command line flag: `-R name_of_repeat_file.gtf`]

   - It is strongly recommended to specify a repetitive region file in GTF format for filtering.

   - A suitable file can for example be obtained through the UCSC table browser: After choosing the genome, a group like **Repeats** or **Variation and Repeats** has to be selected. For the track, we recommend to choose **RepeatMasker** together with **Simple Repeats** and combine the results afterwards. (*See* **Note 1** for additional information.)

3. For paired-end sequencing two files are required, e.g., mate1. txt and mate2.txt which contain the paths to the `chimeric. out.junction` files originating from the separate mate mapping step. [Command line flags: `-m1 mate1.txt and -m2 mate2.txt`]

4. A list of all source BAM files containing the actual reads from the paired-end mapping step has to be prepared. If not specified via the `-B` flag DCC will try to guess their location based on the supplied `chimeric.out.junction` paths. [Command line flag: `-B @bam_files.txt`]

5. The software additionally requires the `SJ.out.tab` files generated by STAR. The program assumes that these files are located in the same folder as the BAM files supplied via `-B`.

6. DCC can be used to process circRNA detection and host gene expression detection either in a one-pass strategy or might be used for only one part of the analysis:

   • Detect circRNAs and host gene expression in one pass: `-D` and `-G` option combined.

   • Detection of circRNAs only: `-D`.

   • Detection of host gene expression only: `-G`.

DCC supports different sequencing protocols widely used for whole-transcriptome experiments. Generally, the user has the option to select between the stranded and unstranded input data (by using the `-N` flag, stranded mode is the default). That is, for a stranded library DCC is able to distinguish if a circRNA is located on the sense or antisense strand. If the sequencing library was prepared in unstranded manner, DCC assigns the strand of the circular based on the host gene's strand since the aligned reads do not provide strand-specific information. Additionally, DCC allows the user to select the library preparation type based on the technique employed—either "firststrand" or "secondstrand" (by using the `-ss` flag). Which option is the correct one depends on the employed sequencing protocol. The following list gives an overview of common sequencing kits and the respective parameter choice:

First-strand kits (default):

• All dUTP methods, NSR, NNSR

• TruSeq Stranded Total RNA Sample Prep Kit

• TruSeq Stranded mRNA Sample Prep Kit

• NEB Ultra Directional RNA Library Prep Kit

• Agilent SureSelect Strand-Specific

Second-strand kits (second-strand parameter -ss has to be used):

- Directional Illumina (Ligation), Standard SOLiD
- ScriptSeq v2 RNA-Seq Library Preparation Kit
- SMARTer Stranded Total RNA
- Encore Complete RNA-Seq Library Systems

Once all input files have been prepared, DCC can be started with the previously generated input files:

```
# Option 1: Running DCC to detect circRNAs in paired
end data
>  DCC @samplesheet \ # @ is generally used to specify
a file name
-mt1 @mate1 \ # mate1 file containing the mate1 inde-
pendently mapped chimeric.junction.out files
-mt2 @mate2 \ # mate2 file containing the mate1 inde-
pendently mapped chimeric.junction.out files
-D \ # run in circRNA detection mode
-R [Repeats].gtf \ # regions in this GTF file are
masked from circRNA detection
-an [Annotation].gtf \ # annotation is used to assign
gene names to known transcripts
-Pi \ # run in paired independent mode, i.e. use -mt1
and -mt2
-F \ # filter the circRNA candidate regions
-M \ # filter out candidates from mitochondrial chromo-
somes
-Nr 5 6 \ minimum number of replicates the candidate
is showing in [1] and minimum count in the replicate
[2]
-fg \ # candidates are not allowed to span more than
one gene
-G \ # also run host gene expression
-A [Reference].fa \ # name of the fasta genome ref-
erence file; must be indexed, i.e. a .fai file must be
present
# Option 2: DCC setup for single end, non-stranded
data:
>  DCC @samplesheet -D -R [Repeats].gtf -an
[Annotation].gtf -F -M -Nr 5 6 -fg -G -A [Reference].fa
>  DCC @samplesheet -mt1 @mate1 -mt2 @mate2 -D -S -R
[Repeats].gtf -an [Annotation].gtf -Pi -F -M -Nr 5 6 -fg
# For details on the parameters please refer to the
help page of DCC:
>  DCC -h
```

The output of DCC consists of the following four files:

- **CircRNACount:** A table containing read counts for circRNAs detected. The first three columns are chromosome, circRNA start, and circRNA end. Starting from the fourth column the circRNA read counts are stored, one sample per column, shown in the order given in the sample sheet.

- **CircCoordinates:** CircRNA annotations in BED format. The columns are chromosome, start coordinate, end coordinate, gene name, junction type (based on STAR; 0: noncanonical; 1: GT/AG, 2: CT/AC, 3: GC/AG, 4: CT/GC, 5: AT/AC, 6: GT/AT), strand, circRNA region (start region–end region), and overall regions (list of genomic features the circRNA coordinate interval covers).

- **LinearCount:** A host gene expression count table with the exact same columns as the CircRNACount file.

- **CircSkipJunctions:** A TSV-based file containing circle skipping junctions. The first three columns are the same as in LinearCount/CircRNACount; the following columns represent the circSkip junctions found for each sample. circSkip junctions are given as chr:start-end:count, e.g., chr1:1787–6949:10. It is possible that for one circRNA multiple circSkip junctions are found due to the fact that the CircRNA may arise from different isoforms. In this case, multiple circSkip junctions are delimited by a semicolon. A 0-entry implies that no circSkip junctions have been found for this specific circRNA and the corresponding library.

3.6 Test for Host: Independently Regulated circRNAs with CircTest

CircTest is optimized for use with DCC-detected circRNAs and thus able to directly work with DCC's output files. CircTest is an R package that can easily be installed for the current user via the R command line:

```
> install.packages("devtools")
> require(devtools)
> install_github('dieterich-lab/CircTest')
> library(CircTest)
```

Since the R package itself is not able to perform analyses, it has to be used within an R script to perform its actual task. A sample R script, working on the RNase R+ and RNase R− data from SRP071584, can be found in the supplementary GitHub repository:

```
https://github.com/dieterich-lab/circular-rna-book/
blob/master/CircTest.R
```

The script may be either called from within R or just directly executed with the Rscript binary:

```
> Rscript CircTest.R
```

The script assumes that the DCC output files are in the same folder as the script. The CircTest script produces an Excel file containing the top 100 enriched circRNAs when comparing RNase R+ and RNase R− samples. Additionally, a PDF file with bar graphs for the top ten circRNAs will be generated.

3.7 Full Circle Characterization with FUCHS

Similar to CircTest, FUCHS is able to directly employ output files generated by DCC. For this part of the work flow the long RNA-seq data from SRP097141 is used to fully exploit FUCHS' ability to reconstruct circRNA sequences. It is assumed that all previous steps (FlexBar, bowtie2, STAR, and DCC) have been performed on the dataset for the FUCHS example. The STAR output has to be slightly preprocessed for FUCHS in that the separate mate mappings have to be merged:

```
# create an index for both BAM files
> samtools index sample_1_mate1.bam
> samtools index sample_1_mate2.bam
# merge both mate BAM files into one new BAM file
> samtools merge sample_1_mate1.bam sample_1_mate2.bam
sample_1_merged_mates.bam
# re-index the newly aggregated BAM file
> samtools index sample_1_merged_mates.bam
```

After merging both separate mate BAM files FUCHS can be installed in a straightforward way via:

```
> git clone git@github.com:dieterich-lab/FUCHS.git
> cd FUCHS
> python setup.py install --user
# This will install a FUCHS binary in $HOME/.local/
bin/
# make sure this folder is in your $PATH
# Check the installation:
> FUCHS --help
```

FUCHS additionally needs an annotation file in BED6 format, which contains exon information for the corresponding genome. A sample file for the mouse mm10 build is provided through the supplementary Git repository:

```
> wget https://github.com/dieterich-lab/circular-
rna-book/blob/master/data/mm10.ensembl.exons.bed.
bz2?raw=true
> bunzip mm10.ensembl.exons.bed.bz2
```

BED files for other species may be obtained through the UCSC genome browser via http://genome.ucsc.edu/cgi-bin/

hgTables by selecting the appropriate organism and choosing BED as output format. On the next page "Create one BED record per: Exon" should be selected.

Once FUCHS has been installed and all required files have been prepared, the tool may be executed using the following parameters:

```
# Run FUCHS main program
> FUCHS -C /path/to/dcc/output/CircRNACount
-J /path/to/sample1/sample1.Chimeric.out.junction
-F /path/to/sample1_mate1/sample_1_mate1.Chimeric.out.
junction
-R /path/to/sample1_mate2/sample_1_mate2.Chimeric.out.
junction. fixed
-B sample_1_merged_mates.bam
-A mm10.ensembl.exons.bed
-r 4
-q 2
-p ensembl
-e 2
-N sample1
-O experiment_X/
# Run FUCHS circRNA reconstruction module
> guided_denovo_circle_structure_parallel -c 4 -A
mm10.ensembl.exons.bed -I experiment_1/ -N sample1
```

Where $-r$ specifies the minimum number of covering reads; $-q$ the minimal mapping quality; $-p$ the reference used for annotation, i.e., either "refseq" or "ensembl"; and $-e$ specifies the appropriate exon id position in the transcript name (3 for refseq, 2 for ensembl). The circRNA list from DCC is provided via $-C$ CircRNACount, the first mate's junction file is specified via $-F$ Chimeric.out.junction, while the second mate's flag is $-R$ Chimeric.out.junction.fixed. The other arguments include the merged BAM file generated in the previous step ($-B$), the annotation file ($-A$), the sample name ($-N$), and the output folder where data should be generated ($-O$).

In order to obtain a more refined circle reconstruction based on intron signals additionally the module guided_denovo_circle_structure_parallel can be executed. The circRNA-separated BAM files generated in the second step are the only input required. If an annotation file is supplied unsupported exons will be reported with a score of 0; otherwise unsupported exons (i.e., no supporting mapping reads) will not be reported.

The output generated by FUCHS consists of several output files which bundle the information gathered during the run. The following list describes the files and their contents (a complete description may be found in the FUCHS repository https:// github.com/dieterich-lab/FUCHS):

- **sample_1/:** Project folder containing all files generated by FUCHS.

- **sample_1.coverage_pictures:** Automatically generated PDF files containing a visual representation of all circRNAs.

- **sample_1.coverage_profiles:** Automatically generated PDF files containing a visual representation of all circRNAs.

- **sample_1.alternative_splicing.txt:** This file summarizes the relationship of different circRNAs derived from the same host gene.

- **sample_1.exon_counts.bed:** This file is a BED-formatted file that describes the exon structure and can be loaded into any genome browser. Each line corresponds to a circRNA.

- **sample_1.exon_counts.txt:** This file contains similar information as the previous file, just more detailed information on the exons. Each line corresponds to one exon.

- **sample_1.mate_status.txt:** This output file contains the results of analyzing the amount of how often each fragment spans a chimeric junction. A fragment can either span the chimeric junction once (single), only one end spans the junction, twice (double) both ends span the chimeric junction, or neither of both (undefined).

- **sample_1.skipped_exons.bed:** A BED12-based file containing skipped exons.

- **sample_1.skipped_exons.txt:** Similar to the BED-based skip file but also contains read information and other details.

- **sample_1_exon_chain_inferred_12.bed:** Output generated by the *de novo* reconstruction script in BED12 format, viewable with any BED-enabled visualization tool.

- **sample_1_exon_chain_inferred_6.bed:** Output generated by the *de novo* reconstruction script in BED6 format, viewable with any BED-enabled visualization tool.

4   Results

4.1   DCC and CircTest

As shown in Fig. 1, the DCC circRNA detection tool functions mainly as a hub, providing raw circRNA counts to be processed by additional downstream tools. In our work flow DCC and CircTest are generally run subsequently as they provide a quick and statistically meaningful overview of the circRNA repertoire in a given experiment (Fig. 2). When used in conjunction with the provided sample R script, the CircTest package generates an Excel-compatible file containing circRNAs that are enriched in the RNase R-treated fraction compared to the mock-treated sample and are statistically significant given an FDR of 0.01. The list does contain not only the position of the circRNA but also the annotation of the respective host gene, thus allowing for fast screen for interesting candidates. Other sub-tables of the file include the raw counts produced by DCC for further in-depth analyses of candidate circRNAs. Additionally to the produced tables, CircTest allows the user to visually assess, e.g., the enrichment of circRNAs. Given the sample R script, CircTest will generate bar graphs for the 100 most significantly enriched circRNAs. Potential other use cases are the comparison of circRNA expression in different tissues, cell lines, or time-course experiments. Especially for time-course experiments the scientist may be able to quickly identify interesting expression patterns.

4.2 Fuchs

FUCHS requires raw counts produced by DCC as well as some additional input files in order to perform analyses. Compared to the data produced by CircTest, FUCHS generates several different output files of different formats for each input circRNA in order to cover a wider range of biological questions. FUCHS works on a per circRNA basis, thus performing its analyses on each input circRNA provided on the command line (usually the circRNAs detected by DCC). In the output folder FUCHS first extracts all sequencing reads belonging to a specific circRNA and stores them in an indexed BAM file which is basis for all further analyses. For deeper inspection these BAM files may be opened with any genome viewer or further processed with samtools. In further steps, FUCHS generates coverage profiles (as plain text) and coverage pictures (in PDF format) for each circRNA. These circRNA-specific files are especially useful when combined with the output from CircTest to further inspect circRNAs of interest without losing the focus on a small subset of candidates. The per-circRNA candidate files are accompanied by whole-experiment files containing results for all input circRNAs including coverage profiles and pictures for the whole circRNA pool as well as a

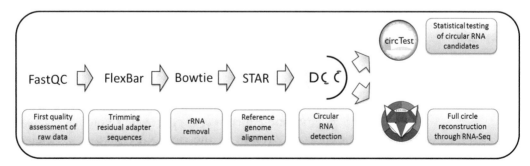

Fig. 1 Overview of the work flow outlined in this manuscript. Several programs are employed for data preprocessing, including FastQC (quality assessment), FlexBar (adapter trimming), Bowtie2 (rRNA removal), and STAR (read mapping). The circRNA-specific part of the pipeline is covered by the three tools DCC (circRNA detection), CircTest (statistical testing of DCC data), and FUCHS (sequence reconstruction for detected circRNAs)

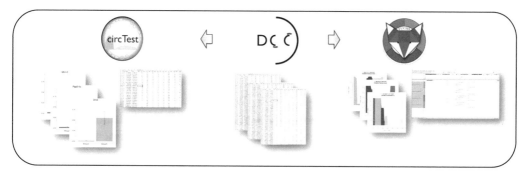

Fig. 2 CircRNA specific part of the work flow focusing data output. DCC is the first program to be executed, generating the raw circRNA counts used by CircTest and FUCHS. CircTest allows for testing of host gene independence (i.e., is the circRNA independently regulated from the host gene) or the comparison of RNase R+ and RNase R− samples in order to estimate the enrichment in the treated sample. CircTest provides output in the form of circRNA lists accompanied by p-value and FDR as well as graphical representations of statistically significant circRNAs. FUCHS is also able to directly employ DCC output to generate coverage profiles and BED tracks for each circRNA as well as sample-wide assessment of length distributions and covered circRNAs

clustering of the circRNAs by length in different categories (short, medium, and long). These accumulated and clustered profiles are very helpful in order to detect any biases in the analyses as those frequently show up as unusual coverage profiles (e.g., circRNAs only covered on one site of the break point). FUCHS is able to provide information on alternative splicing since it is frequent that different circRNAs are originating from the same host gene. Given the mouse sample used throughout this work flow, the amount of host genes having more than one associated circle is around 50% while the most prominent multicircular RNAs share either the same start or end site (which is in agreement with observations of regulatory elements in neighboring introns). To further emphasize the visual component of in silico circRNA research the tool provides a BED file with all circRNAs and their corresponding exon structure which may be viewed in all compatible genome browsers. Additionally, a more detailed plain-text version of the BED file is available that contains information not compatible with the BED format. Complementary to the BED files covering the exons that are part of the circle, FUCHS also generates a BED and plain-text file containing all exons that have been skipped and are not part of the circle. This information allows for example to detect isoforms of circles not yet known as linear isoform of the host gene (which normally is the case). Deeper inspection of the mate pair information (i.e., which part of the mate pair is mapping where in a circle) delivered by FUCHS allows to estimate the length of the detected circRNAs (e.g., ~430 bp in the mouse liver sample). The mate information also allows us to observe a negative correlation of double-breakpoint fragments and circle length. As the name suggests, FUCHS is able to provide information about the complete circRNA which also includes the reconstruction of the circle structure in a guided (using the provided annotation) or de novo fashion. Given our experimental sequencing setup (2 × 250bp reads), FUCHS is able to fully reconstruct circRNAs up to a length of roughly 500 bp which already covers a large portion of the pool of detected circRNAs. The reconstructed circRNAs are again provided as BED files and may be displayed (along with other tracks) in all common genome browsers.

5   Notes

1. DCC Repeat File Conversion

   The obtained repeat file needs to comply with the GTF format specification. Additionally it may be the case that the names of chromosomes from different databases differ, e.g., 1 for chromosome 1 from ENSEMBL compared to chr1 for chromosome 1 from UCSC. Since the chromosome names are important for the correct functionality of DCC a sample command for converting the identifiers may be:

```
# Example to convert UCSC identifiers to to ENSEMBL
standard
> sed -i 's/^chr//g' repeat_file.gtf
```

Acknowledgments

Both authors acknowledge funding by the Klaus Tschira Foundation gGmbH.

References

1. Hoffmann S et al (2014) A multi-split mapping algorithm for circular RNA, splicing, trans-splicing and fusion detection. Genome Biol 15(2):R34

2. Wang K et al (2010) MapSplice: accurate mapping of RNA-seq reads for splice junction discovery. Nucleic Acids Res 38(18):1–14

3. Memczak S et al (2013) Circular RNAs are a large class of animal RNAs with regulatory potency. Nature 495(7441):333–338

4. Chuang TJ, Wu CS, Chen CY, Hung LY, Chiang TW, Yang MY (2015) NCLscan: accurate identification of non-co-linear transcripts (fusion, trans-splicing and circular RNA) with a good balance between sensitivity and precision. Nucleic Acids Res 44(3):e29

5. Dodt M, Roehr JT, Ahmed R, Dieterich C (2012) FLEXBAR—flexible barcode and adapter processing for next-generation sequencing platforms. Biology (Basel) 1(3):895–905

6. Westholm JO et al (2014) Genome-wide analysis of drosophila circular RNAs reveals their structural and sequence properties and age-dependent neural accumulation. Cell Rep 9(5):1966–1981

7. Zhang XO, Bin Wang H, Zhang Y, Lu X, Chen LL, Yang L (2014) Complementary sequence-mediated exon circularization. Cell 159(1):134–147

8. Gao Y, Wang J, Zhao F (2015) CIRI: an efficient and unbiased algorithm for de novo circular RNA identification. Genome Biol 16(1):4

9. Cheng J, Metge F, Dieterich C (2016) Specific identification and quantification of circular RNAs from sequencing data. Bioinformatics 32(7):1094–1096

10. Szabo L et al (2015) Statistically based splicing detection reveals neural enrichment and tissue-specific induction of circular RNA during human fetal development. Genome Biol 16:126

11. Dobin A et al (2013) STAR: ultrafast universal RNA-seq aligner. Bioinformatics 29(1):15–21

12. Langmead B, Salzberg SL (2012) Fast gapped-read alignment with Bowtie 2. Nat Methods 9(4):357–360

13. Li H, Durbin R (2009) Fast and accurate short read alignment with Burrows-Wheeler transform. Bioinformatics 25(14):1754–1760

14. Jeck WR, Sharpless NE (2014) Detecting and characterizing circular RNAs. Nat Biotechnol 32(5):453–461

15. Metge F, Czaja-Hasse LF, Reinhardt R, Dieterich C (2017) FUCHS—towards full circular RNA characterization using RNAseq. PeerJ 5:e2934

16. Li H et al (Aug. 2009) The sequence alignment/map format and SAMtools. Bioinformatics 25(16):2078–2079

17. R Core Team (2013) R: a language and environment for statistical computing. Vienna, Austria

18. Andrews S (2012) FastQC. A Qual. Control tool high throughput Seq. data. [http//www.bioinformatics.bbsrc.ac.uk/projects/fastqc/]

19. Jakobi T, Czaja-Hasse LF, Reinhardt R, Dieterich C (2016) Profiling and validation of the circular RNA repertoire in adult murine hearts. Genomics, Proteomics Bioinforma 14(4):216–223

Chapter 3

Genome-Wide circRNA Profiling from RNA-seq Data

Daphne A. Cooper, Mariela Cortés-López, and Pedro Miura

Abstract

The genome-wide expression patterns of circular RNAs (circRNAs) are of increasing interest for their potential roles in normal cellular homeostasis, development, and disease. Thousands of circRNAs have been annotated from various species in recent years. Analysis of publically available or user-generated rRNA-depleted total RNA-seq data can be performed to uncover new circRNA expression trends. Here we provide a primer for profiling circRNAs from RNA-seq datasets. The description is tailored for the wet lab scientist with limited or no experience in analyzing RNA-seq data. We begin by describing how to access and interpret circRNA annotations. Next, we cover converting circRNA annotations into junction sequences that are used as scaffolds to align RNA-seq reads. Lastly, we visit quantifying circRNA expression trends from the alignment data.

Key words circRNA, Circular RNAs, Expression analysis, Ribo-depleted total RNA-seq

1 Introduction

Detection of circRNAs in RNA-seq data is limited to stranded, ribosomal RNA (rRNA/ribo)-depleted total RNA-seq, as opposed to library preparation protocols requiring enrichment of polyadenylated RNAs. Total RNA-seq libraries are becoming increasingly common since they detect a variety of RNAs, including both mRNAs and non-polyadenylated RNAs. Over the past few years, thousands of circRNAs have been annotated in humans, mice, fish, insects, plants, and yeast from total RNA-seq data, using algorithms designed to detect "out-of-order" splicing [1–12]. These analysis pipelines include find_circ [2], circRNA_finder [8], CIRCexplorer [13], and CIRI [14], among others [15, 16]. Most of these algorithms and analysis pipelines can detect exonic, intronic, and intergenic circRNAs, whereas CIRCfinder is a pipeline designed to exclusively detect intronic circRNAs [17]. Despite thousands of circRNA annotations, novel circRNAs continue to be annotated, and the user should consider that specific tissues or cell types of interest might express novel circRNAs that necessitate the use of one of the previously mentioned circRNA detection algorithms.

Christoph Dieterich and Argyris Papantonis (eds.), *Circular RNAs: Methods and Protocols*, Methods in Molecular Biology, vol. 1724, https://doi.org/10.1007/978-1-4939-7562-4_3, © Springer Science+Business Media, LLC 2018

It is generally required that the total RNA-seq datasets to be analyzed for circRNA expression trends are of very high depth, due to only circRNA junction spanning reads being used in the analysis. CircRNA junction spanning reads typically comprise less than 0.1% of the reads generated in a total RNA-seq experiment [5].

Here, we provide a primer for profiling circRNAs from RNA-seq datasets using existing circRNA annotations. Table 1 provides a reference for reports and online databases containing circRNA

Table 1 circRNA annotations

Annotations in reports			
Organism	**Genome annotation**	**Conditions**	**References**
Mus musculus	mm9	Brain; synaptoneurosomes; liver; heart; embryonic stem cell neuronal diff.; P19 cell neuronal diff.; primary neuron diff.	[2–5]
Homo sapiens	hg19	Brain; SH-SY5Y cell neuronal diff.; HEK293 cells; CD34+ cells; CD19+ cells; neutrophils; Hs68 cells; DLD-1 cells; DKO-1 cells, DKs-8 cells	[1, 2, 4, 32, 33]
Drosophila melanogaster	dm3	Heads; S2 cells	[3, 8]
Caenorhabditis elegans	ce6	Various tissues and developmental stages	[2, 34]

Annotations in online databases			
Database name	**Web address**	**Description**	**References**
circBase	www.circbase.org	circRNAs from various tissues, cell types, and developmental stages from human, mouse, fruit fly, *C. elegans*, and others	[35]
circRNAdb	http://reprod.njmu.edu.cn/circrnadb	Human circRNAs by cell type, protein-coding potential, gene symbol and PubMed ID	[36]
CircNet	http://circnet.mbc.nctu.edu.tw	Human tissue-specific circRNA expression information and miRNA binding potential	[37]
Tissue-specific circRNA database	http://gb.whu.edu.cn/TSCD	Human and mouse circRNA from various tissues	[38]

annotations from various organisms. In this example, a circRNA annotation set is used to generate a circRNA junction scaffold Bowtie2 aligner index. Reads that align to the circRNA junction scaffold are summed using featureCounts and the number of reads that align to each circRNA junction is normalized to the read depth of the library. This normalization allows the direct comparison of circRNA expression from different conditions so that differentially expressed circRNAs can be identified.

2   Materials

1. Computer running Linux or Mac OSX.

2. UNIX shell (e.g., bash).

3. Installed open-access software:

    (a) Bedtools [18]: github.com/arq5x/bedtools2/releases.

    (b) Bowtie2 [19]: bowtie-bio.sourceforge.net/bowtie2/index.shtml.

    (c) Samtools [20, 21]: samtools. sourceforge.net.

    (d) featureCounts [22]: subread.sourceforge.net.

4. rRNA-depleted total RNA-seq data in FASTQ format (user generated or downloaded from repository).

5. Genome sequence for species of interest in FASTA format.

6. circRNA annotations for species of interest in BED6 format.

7. *Optional*: Integrative Genomics Viewer (IGV) [23, 24].

8. *Optional*: SRAtools: github.com/ncbi/sra-tools.

3   Methods

3.1   Generate circRNA Junction Sequences

1. *View contents of a circRNA annotation BED file.* Many circRNA annotations are provided as a list of genomic coordinates or as Browser Extensible Data (BED) records that describe the genomic coordinates and other information (https://genome.ucsc.edu/FAQ/FAQformat#format1). The BED format includes a chromosome (chrom), a 0-based start (chromStart) position in base pair units, a stop position (chromStop), a feature name, a score, and strand information (Fig. 1a). The score can provide information about the expression level of a particular circRNA; however it is often assigned a "0" value. The strand assignment provides information about whether the circRNA is encoded from the sense or antisense DNA strand. Figure 1a illustrates a BED file (circRNA.bed) that contains annotations for two circRNAs (circ_1 and circ_2). The BED annotation is used to generate junction sequences

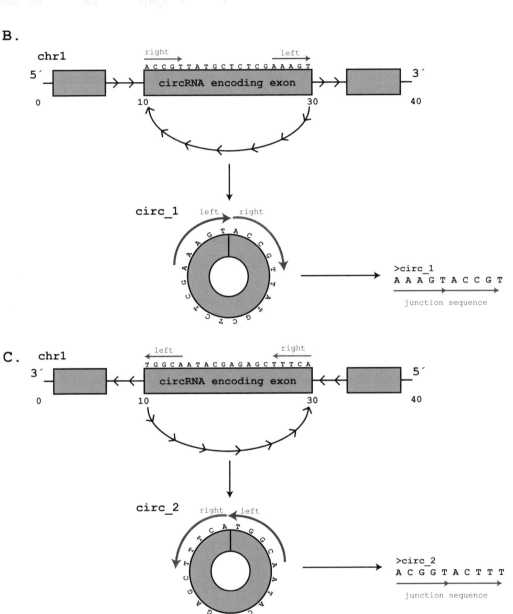

A.

chrom	chromStart	chromStop	name	score	strand
chr1	10	30	**circ_1**	0	+
chr1	10	30	**circ_2**	0	–
chr1	50	37	circ_3	0	–
chr2	200	310	circ_4	0	+

B.

chr1

right   left

A C C G T T A T G C T C T C G A A A G T

circRNA encoding exon

circ_1

left   right

>circ_1
A A A G T A C C G T

junction sequence

C.

chr1

left   right

T G G C A A T A C G A G A G C T T T C A

circRNA encoding exon

circ_2

right   left

>circ_2
A C G G T A C T T T

junction sequence

Fig. 1 circRNA junction formation from BED annotations. (**a**) Representative BED file, circRNA.bed, a tab-delimited file that reports the chromosomal location and features of circRNAs. (**b**) Model of a 3-exon protein-coding gene with exon 2 encoding a circRNA. circ_1 maps to chr1 from nt 10 to 30. The downstream "left" end of the exon (at nt 30) joins with the upstream "right" end of the exon to form the circRNA junction. (**c**) circ_2 is encoded on the antisense DNA strand, but has the same start and stop coordinates as circ_1. The upstream "left" side of the exon joins with the downstream "right" side of the exon to form the circRNA junction. Because circ_2 is encoded on the antisense DNA strand, the sequence is reverse-complemented relative to circ_1. FASTA-formatted junction sequences (Subheading 3.1, **step 4**) are used to build the aligner index (Subheading 3.2, **step 1**) necessary for alignment of RNA-seq data to circRNA junctions (Subheading 3.2)

circ_1 (Fig. 1b) and circ_2 (Fig. 1c). Both circ_1 and circ_2 are 20 nucleotides (nts) in length, and have the same genomic coordinates; however, circ_1 is encoded on the sense DNA strand and circ_2 is encoded on the antisense DNA strand to highlight how strand orientation impacts the directionality and sequence of circRNAs. CircRNAs encoded on the sense strand of DNA are assigned a "+" in the sixth "strand" field (Fig. 1a: circ_1), while those encoded on the antisense DNA strand are assigned a "−" (Fig. 1a: circ_2). Genes encoded on the antisense DNA strand run 3′ to 5′ in relation to the sense strand; therefore the chromStop field represents the "start" of the gene, and the chromStart field represents the "stop" of the gene. Because circ_2 is encoded on the antisense DNA strand, it is reverse complemented in relation to circ_1 (Fig. 1c). Note that 10 nt junction sequences for circ_1 and circ_2 join the last 5 nts with the first 5 nts of the circularizing exon and run in the 5′–3′ direction (Fig. 1b, c; **junction sequence**).

For this primer on circRNA expression profiling, we used the first four records in the mouse cortex annotation from Supplemental Table 2 in Gruner et al. (2016) [5], to make cortex_circRNA.bed. These four BED records will be used to generate circRNA junction sequences of 200 nt length in the manner illustrated in Fig. 1.

```
# View contents of cortex_circRNA.bed

$ more cortex_circRNA.bed

chrX    58436422   58439349    CDR1as            0    +
chr1    154691165  154691537   mm9_circ_000025   0    -
chr1    16430403   16453275    mm9_circ_000040   0    -
chr18   51462263   51463167    mm9_circ_000042   0    +
```

2. *Split the annotations into circRNAs encoded from the sense "+" strand and circRNAs encoded from the antisense "−" strand.* Write circRNAs encoded on the "+" strand to a file named "sense. cortex_circRNA.bed" and write circRNAs encoded on the "−" strand to a file named "antisense.cortex_circRNA.bed".

```
$ awk '($6 == "+")' cortex_circRNA.bed > sense.cortex_circRNA.bed
$ awk '($6 == "-")' cortex_circRNA.bed > antisense.cortex_circRNA.bed
```

3. *Modify the BED start and stop coordinates to represent half the length of the desired junction scaffold sequence for the "left" and "right" sides of the circRNA junction* (Fig. 1b, c). For this example, we generate a junction of 200 nts in length to accommodate RNA-seq reads of 125 nts in length [5]. Using these conditions, an end-to-end Bowtie2 alignment would at minimum require at least a 25-nt overlap of the circRNA

junction. RNA-seq data generated from the Illumina platform will generally range in length from 50 to 150 nts. When using real RNA-seq data, consider the junction overlap, and choose a junction scaffold length that will accommodate the read length of your RNA-seq data.

The desired junction scaffold length for this example is 200 nts in length; therefore, the start and stop coordinates reported in the modified BED annotation for the "left" (Fig. 1b, c; blue arrows) and "right" (Fig. 1b, c; red arrows) sides of the junction will be 100 nts in length (half of the total junction scaffold length). The 100-nt "left" and "right" sequences will be joined to form the out-of-order circRNA junction scaffold sequence similar to the junctions depicted in Fig. 1b, c. For circRNAs encoded on the "+" strand, the "chromStop" position is used to generate the "left" side of the circRNA junction by subtracting 100 nts from the chromStop position, and then writing a new BED record to a file called "l_junc.sense.cortex_circRNA.bed" to represent the 100-nt left half of the junction. For the right side of the junction, 100 nts are added to the chromStart position, and the BED record is written to a file called "r_junc.sense.cortex_circRNA.bed" to represent the 100-nt right half of the junction. For circRNAs encoded on the "−" strand, the "chromStart" position is used to generate the "left" side of the circRNA junction by adding 100 nts to the chromStart position, and then writing the BED record to a file called "l_junc.antisense.cortex_circRNA.bed" to represent the 100-nt left half of the junction. For the right side of the junction, 100 nts are subtracted from the chromStop position, and the BED record is written to a file called "r_junc.antisense.cortex_circRNA.bed" to represent the 100-nt right side of the junction. There are some limitations with capturing circRNAs that are smaller than the desired circRNA junction scaffold length (*see* **Note 1**):

```
$ awk 'OFS="\t" {$2=$3-100} {print $0}' sense.cortex_circRNA.bed \
    > l_junc.sense.cortex_circRNA.bed

$ awk 'OFS="\t" {$3=$2+100} {print $0}' sense.cortex_circRNA.bed \
    > r_junc.sense.cortex_circRNA.bed

$ awk 'OFS="\t" {$3=$2+100} {print $0}' antisense.cortex_circRNA.bed \
    > l_junc.antisense.cortex_circRNA.bed

$ awk 'OFS="\t" {$2=$3-100} {print $0}' antisense.cortex_circRNA.bed \
    > r_junc.antisense.cortex_circRNA.bed
```

4. *Extract the "left" and "right" 100-nt sequences that will form the circRNA junction with the bedtools "getfasta" subcommand.* Both a BED file (generated in the previous step) and a FASTA file containing the appropriate genome sequence are required to build the junction scaffold with the bedtools "getfasta" subcommand.

Ensure that the annotations in the BED and genome FASTA file have the same chromosome name. iGenomes and Ensembl annotate genome FASTA chromosomes as a number only, whereas UCSC genome browser includes a "chr" prefix prior to the chromosome number (e.g., 1 vs. chr1). FASTA files of the genome or different genomes of interest organized by chromosome or contigs can be downloaded directly from

UCSC Genome Browser: http://hgdownload.cse.ucsc.edu/downloads.html.

Ensembl: ftp://ftp.ensembl.org/pub/release-87/fasta/.

Illumina iGenomes: support.illumina.com/sequencing/sequencing_software/igenome.html.

```
# Extract sequences for "left" and "right" sides of circRNA junctions for
circRNAs encoded on "+" strand.
$ bedtools getfasta -fi mm9.genome.fa -bed l_junc.sense.cortex_circRNA.bed \
     -s -name -tab -fo l_junc.sense.cortex_circRNA.seq

$ bedtools getfasta -fi mm9.genome.fa -bed r_junc.sense.cortex_circRNA.bed \
     -s -name -tab -fo r_junc.sense.cortex_circRNA.seq

# Extract sequences for "left" and "right" sides of circRNA junctions for
circRNAs encoded on the "-" strand.
$ bedtools getfasta -fi mm9.genome.fa -bed l_junc.antisense.cortex_circRNA.bed \
     -s -name -tab -fo l_junc.antisense.cortex_circRNA.seq

$ bedtools getfasta -fi mm9.genome.fa -bed r_junc.antisense.cortex_circRNA.bed \
     -s -name -tab -fo r_junc.antisense.cortex_circRNA.seq
```

5. *Combine the "left" and "right" sequences to form the 200-nt junction scaffold sequence in FASTA format.* The FASTA output for the circRNA junctions is shown in Fig. 2.

```
$ paste l_junc.sense.cortex_circRNA.seq r_junc.sense.cortex_circRNA.seq \
     | awk '{print ">"$1"\n"$2$4}' > circRNA_junctions.fa

# Append "-" strand circRNA junction sequence to "circRNA_junction.fa"
$ paste l_junc.antisense.cortex_circRNA.seq r_junc.antisense.cortex_circRNA.seq \
     | awk '{print">"$1"\n"$2$4}' >> circRNA_junctions.fa
```

3.2 Align RNA-seq Reads to the circRNA Junction Scaffold

1. *Build the Bowtie2 aligner index using the circRNA junction scaffold.* Six index files with the extension .bt2 are generated by bowtie2-build.

   ```
   $ bowtie2-build circRNA_junctions.fa circRNA_junctions
   ```

2. *Obtain RNA-seq datasets in FASTQ format if user-generated RNA-seq data is not available.* Ensure that the library strategy used to generate the RNA-seq data is rRNA-depleted total RNA-seq. Publicly available RNA-seq datasets are available on

```
$ more circRNA_junctions.fa
>CDR1as
TCCACATCTTCCAGCATCTTTATGTCTTCCAACAACTGCGCAGTGTCTCCAGTGTATCGGCGTTTTGACATTCAGGTTTTCTGGTGTCTGCCGTATCCAG
GGTTTCCAGTGGTGCCAGTACCAAGGTCTTCCAACATCTCCAGGTCTTCCAGCAACTGCAAGTCTTCCAACACTGTCAAGGTCTTCCAGACAATCGTGAT
>mm9_circ_000042
ATAAACGTAAAATAATAAGTAATGAGCACTTTCTACTCAAGCAATAAAAAGCCCAAATATATTAATCTGCATTCAACAAAGTGGCATAAAAAATCACGTG
GTGGTTGACCAGATTGACACCCTGACCTCTGATCTACAGCTGGAAGATGAGATGACCGACAGCTCCAAAACAGACACTCTGAACAGCAGCTCCAGTGGGA
>mm9_circ_000025
AGCAGTAATGGCTCAGCAACCAAATATGGACCGCAGGAGCAAACGGTCACCTGGAGTCTTCCGTCCAGAACAGGATCCTGTGCCCAGGATGCCATTTGAG
TATCAACAGGCAGATGCCTCCAAACAGCTGTGGAATCCCCCTCAGGTTCAAAGCCCACTAGGGAAAATTATGCCTGTGAAACAGTCCTACTACCTTCAGA
>mm9_circ_000040
CTATGAAAAGGGGAGAGCCTGCCATCTACAGGCCACTAGATCCAAAGCCATTCCCAAATTATAGAGCTAACTACAACTTCCGGGGCATGTACAATCAGAG
ATGTTTTCGGTGCAGCTGAGTCTTGGCGAGCAGACATGGGAATCCGAAGGGAGCAGTATAAAGAAGGCCCAACAAGCTGTTGCTAACAAAGCTTTGACTG
```

Fig. 2 circRNA junction FASTA sequences. The resulting 200 nt circRNA junction sequences in FASTA format after joining the 100-nt "left" and "right" sequences (Subheading 3.1, **step 5**)

ENCODE: www.encodeproject.org

NCBI Gene Expression Omnibus (GEO): http://www.ncbi.nlm.nih.gov/geo

NCBI Sequence Record Archive (SRA): http://www.ncbi.nlm.nih.gov/sra

SRAtools (https://github.com/ncbi/sra-tools) is needed to extract FASTQ data from SRA files downloaded from GEO and SRA. Obtain at least two RNA-seq datasets from different conditions to compare changes in circRNA expression. For the purposes of this example, we use the SRA prefetch tool to obtain total RNA/rRNA-depleted RNA-seq datasets deposited on the SRA for two conditions: one replicate each for 1-month-old (SRR4280863) mouse cortex and 22-month-old (SRR4280956) mouse cortex [5]. Once the SRA files have been downloaded, the SRA tool fastq-dump is used to extract the FASTQ files from the SRA files. Since these RNA-seq datasets are paired end, the read 1 data are contained in the "_1.fastq.gz" file and the read 2 data are contained in the "_2.fastq.gz" file. Both the read 1 and read 2 files will have the same number of records, and each record will have the same read ID (Fig. 3). The quality of the datasets can be assessed using FastQC (*see* **Note 2**):

```
#use the prefetch tool from the SRA toolkit to download datasets from the SRA
#The downloaded files will have a .sra extension
$ prefetch SRR4280863
$ prefetch SRR4280956

#extract FASTQ data from .sra files and split into read1 and read2 using the SRA
tool fastq-dump
$ fastq-dump --split-files -F --gzip SRR4280863
$ fastq-dump --split-files -F --gzip SRR4280956

#rename datasets
$ mv SRR4280863_1.fastq.gz 1m-cortex.R1.fastq.gz
$ mv SRR4280863_2.fastq.gz 1m-cortex.R2.fastq.gz
$ mv SRR4280956_1.fastq.gz 22m-cortex.R1.fastq.gz
$ mv SRR4280956_2.fastq.gz 22m-cortex.R2.fastq.gz
```

```
$ zcat 1m-cortex.R1.fastq.gz | head -n4
@HWI-D00269:140:C7FJYANXX:3:1101:1083:1885
NTTTGGNNNNNNNNNNNNNNNNNNNNNNNNNNNNNNNNNNNNNNNNNNNNNTANNANTGNACNNNNATNNNNTTTNNNNGTAACCNGCTANNNNCAAGNTNGTTAGNNTTTTCACNNATCGGA
+HWI-D00269:140:C7FJYANXX:3:1101:1083:1885
#<=BBG#########################################--##-#::#--####<-####<<####9<=CFF#;;F@####9;:9#8#::CGG##::9DGE/##68CCED

$ zcat 1m-cortex.R2.fastq.gz |head -n4
@HWI-D00269:140:C7FJYANXX:3:1101:1083:1885
GTGAAAAGCCTAACGAGCTTGGTGATAGCTGGTTACCCAAAAAATGAATTTAAGTTCAATTTTAAACTTGCTAAAAAAACAACAAAATCAAAAAGTAAGTTTAGATTATAGCCAAAAAGATCGGA
+HWI-D00269:140:C7FJYANXX:3:1101:1083:1885
BBBCCGGGGGGGGGGGGGGGGGGGGGGGGGGGGGGGGGGGGGGGF GGGGGGGGGGGGGGGGGGGGGGGGGGF GGGGGGGGGGGGGGGGF GGGGGGGGGGGGGGGGDF GGG>F GGGF GGGGGGGGGEGGGG
```

Fig. 3 FASTQ records in read 1 and read 2 RNA-seq datasets. Each sequence record in the FASTQ file is composed of four lines. The first line always begins with an "@" character, followed by the read ID (in this example: HWI-D00269:140:C7FJYANXX:3:1101:1083:1885). The second line of FASTQ record is the read sequence, the third line is a "+" character with or without other read information, and the fourth line contains the sequencing qualities reported for each base. The RNA-seq FASTQ datasets for read 1 (1m-cortex.R1.fastq.gz) and read 2 (1m-cortex.R2.fastq.gz) contain the same number of records and the same read IDs

3. *Align FASTQ datasets to the junction scaffold using Bowtie2.* In this example, we use a minimum alignment score of −15 regardless of read length. Stringency of alignment output can be altered by various parameters in Bowtie2. These parameters are covered in the Bowtie2 manual (http://bowtie-bio.source-forge.net/bowtie2/manual.shtml). By default, Bowtie2 dumps its output to standard out (stdout). However, in this example, stdout is piped to samtools view to write a Binary Alignment Mapping (BAM) output file that includes only mapped reads sorted by the reference sequence and leftmost alignment position. BAM files are compressed binary versions of the Sequence Alignment Mapping (SAM) file. Checking the SAM/BAM alignment reports is critical to ensuring accurate alignment to the circRNA junctions (*see* **Note 3**). The circRNA alignment information provided in the SAM/BAM file is covered in Fig. 4 for the first aligned read reported in 1m-cortex.bam:

```
$ bowtie2 --score-min=C,-15,0 -x circRNA_junctions \
    -1 1m-cortex.R1.fastq.gz -2 1m-cortex.R2.fastq.gz \
    | samtools view -ShuF4 - \
    | samtools sort - -m 8G 1m-cortex

#repeat alignment for second condition
```

3.3 Count Reads that Align to circRNA Junctions Using Featurecounts

1. *Generate a Gene Transfer Format (GTF) file using the cortex_circRNA.bed file that contains the circRNA name information.* The circRNA GTF output is shown in Fig. 5.

```
$ awk '(OFS="\t") \
{print $4, "Gruner_2016", "junction", "1", "200", ".", "+", ".", "circID
\""$4"\""} \
    ' cortex_circRNA.bed > circRNA.gtf
```

```
$ samtools view 1m-cortex.bam | head -n1 | cut -f1-12
HWI-D00269:140:C7FJYANXX:3:1103:10854:76709     163     CDR1as    1    42    125M    =    29    153
TCCACATCTTCCAGCATCTTTATGTCTTCCAACAACTGCGCAGTGTCTCCAGTGTATCGGCGTTTTGACATTCAGGTTTTCTGGTGTCTGCCGTATCCAGGGTTTCCAGTGGTGCCAGTACCAAG
B@BBBGGGGGFCFGG1FGG@GGCFG>@1EFCGGG0GGGGGDCGD1:CFGGCDGEG@GGGG@GB/EBGED1<<EGFG=FG0FGGEGGGC00<<>>8F0C>00;:CGG0D08C0<9C0FGG==0;0:
AS:i:0
```

Fig. 4 1m-cortex.bam output from Bowtie2 alignment for first mapped read. The meaning of fields in SAM/BAM output reports is described at samtools.github.io/hts-specs/. In 1m-cortex.bam, generated from the Bowtie2 alignment (Subheading 3.2, **step 3**), the first reported read is assigned a FLAG value of 163. This FLAG value indicates that the read is properly paired, is the second in the pair, and its mate is reverse complemented relative to the reference. The output also indicates that the read aligns to the CDR1as circRNA junction scaffold reference starting at nt 1 (field 4). The mapping quality (MAPQ) field value is 42, and the entire 125-nt (125M) RNA-seq read aligned to the CDR1as junction. An "=" character is assigned to field 7 to indicate that the mate read aligns to the same reference sequence. Field 8 reports that the mate read aligns at position 29 of the reference sequence. The inferred fragment length of 153 nts from the read1 and read2 alignment is reported in field 9. The sequence and the quality scores for the read are reported in fields 10 and 11, and the alignment score is reported in field 12. A perfect alignment in Bowtie2 end-to-end mode will produce a score of 0, while various alignment penalties (e.g., mismatches, insertions, gaps) will report negative scores

```
$ more circRNA.gtf
CDR1as             Gruner_2016    junction   1    200    .    +    .    circID"CDR1as"
mm9_circ_000025    Gruner_2016    junction   1    200    .    +    .    circID"mm9_circ_000025"
mm9_circ_000040    Gruner_2016    junction   1    200    .    +    .    circID"mm9_circ_000040"
mm9_circ_000042    Gruner_2016    junction   1    200    .    +    .    circID"mm9_circ_000042"
```

Fig. 5 circRNA GTF for featureCounts. The GTF generated in 3.3.1 provides (1) the circRNA name, (2) the source of data, (3) a feature, (4) the start position of the feature (1-based), (5) the end position, (6) the score (can be replaced with a "."), (7) the strand, (8) the frame (can be replaced with a "."), and (9) an attribute, which is a semicolon-separated list of tag-value pairs

2. *Run featureCounts using the BAM files and the newly generated circRNA GTF file as input to count the reads that aligned to each circRNA junction.* Multiple BAM files representing replicates and different conditions can be fed into feature-Counts simultaneously. The featureCounts output is an easy-to-interpret data frame that includes the read count for each circRNA for each condition (Fig. 6):

```
$ featureCounts -C -T 4 -t junction -g circID -a circRNA.gtf -o circRNA.counts.txt \
    1m-cortex.bam 22m-cortex.bam
```

3.4 Normalize circRNA Counts to Compare circRNA Expression Across Conditions

1. *Determine total library size for normalization using transcripts per million (TPM).* TPM is one approach for library normalization [5]. For this normalization approach, total read number generated per library is required. For paired-end RNA-seq libraries, this includes the sum of raw FASTQ records from both the read 1 (.R1.fastq.gz) and read 2 (.R2.fastq.gz) RNA-seq files. In this example, 1m-cortex.R1.fastq.gz includes 51,789,102 records, and 1m-cortex.R2.fastq.gz includes 51,789,102 records; thus, the total size of library is 103,678,204 reads. Because each FASTQ record is made up of

```
$ more circRNA.counts.txt
# Program:featureCounts v1.5.0; Command:"featureCounts" "-C" "-T" "4" "-t" "junction" "-g" "circID"
"-a" "circRNA.gtf" "-o" "circRNA.counts.txt" "1m-cortex.bam" "22m-cortex.bam"
Geneid             Chr              Start   End  Strand Length 1m-cortex.bam  22m-cortex.bam
CDR1as             CDR1as               1   200   +      200    29              45
mm9_circ_000025    mm9_circ_000025      1   200   +      200    11              21
mm9_circ_000040    mm9_circ_000040      1   200   +      200     5               1
mm9_circ_000042    mm9_circ_000042      1   200   +      200     4              16
```

Fig. 6 FeatureCounts output. Output generated from featureCounts (Subheading 3.3, **step 2**) provides the count of reads for each circRNA feature. For example, 29 individual reads aligned to CDR1as circRNA junction in the 1m-cortex sample versus 45 individual reads in the 22m-cortex sample

four lines, the total number of lines in the RNA-seq FASTQ data file divided by four can be used to determine the total library size. In addition, the output log of Bowtie2 reports the total number of reads processed:

```
$ zcat 1m-cortex.R1.fastq.gz | wc -l
207156408
#Number of reads in Read1 FASTQ file: 207156408/4 = 51789102 reads

$ zcat 1m-cortex.R2.fastq.gz | wc -l
207156408
#Number of reads in Read2 FASTQ file: 207156408/4 = 51789102 reads
```

2. *Normalize counts to TPM*. Divide the number of reads that aligned to each circRNA by total library size. The result is multiplied by 1,000,000, and then divided by the scaling factor. The scaling factor is the length of the circRNA junction in kilobases (kb). The junction scaffold used for this example was 200 nts in length; thus the scaling factor is 0.2 kb:

```
$ awk '(NR > 2)' circRNA.counts.txt \
   | awk  -v lib_size_1m=103678204 -v lib_size_22m=102442864 'OFS="\t" \
   {TPM_1m=((( $7/lib_size_1m)*10^6)/0.2)} \
   {TPM_22m=((( $8/lib_size_22m)*10^6)/0.2)} \
   {print $1, TPM_1m, TPM_22m}' \
    > circRNA_TPM.txt

#view normalized data
$ cat circRNA_TPM.txt
CDR1as             1.39856       2.19635
mm9_circ_000025    0.530488      1.02496
mm9_circ_000040    0.241131      0.0488077
mm9_circ_000042    0.192905      0.780923
```

3. *Quantify circRNA expression trends*. Now that the circRNA counts are normalized, the different libraries/conditions can be directly compared. In our example, libraries of cortex RNA from 1-month-old mice have 1.4 TPM for CDR1as versus 2.2 TPM from 22-month-old mice. From here, fold change can be

calculated to determine fluxes in circRNA expression (e.g., a 1.6-fold increase in CDR1as circRNA from 1 m to 22 m). The R base package is useful for performing statistical tests, and can be used in addition to the ggplot2 library for plotting expression changes in circRNAs [25, 26]. Expression trends of circRNAs observed with RNA-seq data should be validated using experimental methods such as RT-qPCR and Northern blot analysis. Additional chapters within this book detail these methodologies to study circRNAs (*see* **Note 4**).

4   Notes

1. A caveat of this method for the generation of junction is that it does not take into account the size of the circRNA. If a circRNA is derived from a single exon that is smaller than the size of the desired junction sequence length, the above script will grab flanking non-circRNA sequence, like introns or intergenic sequence. For circRNAs smaller than the desired junction, options include (1) generating a shorter junction sequence or (2) maintaining the desired length of the junction sequence by concatenating the circRNA sequence. A rough circRNA length can be determined by subtracting the chromStart position from the chromStop position in the BED record.

2. The quality of RNA-seq libraries can be assessed with fastQC (http://www.bioinformatics.babraham.ac.uk/projects/fastqc/). Among the quality measures of fastQC is sequence duplication, or repetitive reads due to PCR duplicates. Although the impact of PCR duplicates on RNA expression is debatable [27–29], PCR duplicates may impact circRNA profiling due to the low frequency of circRNA junction-specific reads. Picard MarkDuplicates (https://github.com/broadinstitute/picard) or samtools rmdup can be used to remove PCR duplicates from alignment BAM files. FastQC also reports adapter contamination in the RNA-seq reads. Adapter contamination occurs if the cDNA insert is shorter than the desired read length, and the adapter sequence or a portion of the adapter sequence is included in the read output. Reads with considerable adapter sequence will not align to the circRNA junction scaffold in Bowtie2 end-to-end mode, so trimming adapter sequence can potentially enhance alignment to the circRNA junction scaffold. An option for trimming adapter sequence is Cutadapt [30]; however, adapter-trimmed sequences will result in variable read length, and filtering the alignments to require circRNA junction overlap will be necessary.

3. Spot check the junction sequences by loading circRNA BED annotations on IGV [23, 24] or UCSC genome browser [31] to ensure that the proper junction is accurately captured. The alignment BAM files can also be loaded onto IGV with the junction scaffold FASTA file (as the genome). A BAM index file (bam.bai) is required for each BAM file loaded onto IGV. To generate the index file, use samtools "index". Visualizing the reads aligned onto the circRNA scaffold through IGV can help the user spot low mapping quality and other systemic errors.

4. As there are a huge number of predicted circRNAs, very few annotations have been validated by independent methods such as Sanger sequencing of circRNA RT-PCR products, RNase R treatment, or Northern blot techniques (see additional chapters in the book). It is important for the user to validate circRNA expression trends using independent molecular techniques.

Acknowledgments

This work was supported by the National Institute of General Medical Sciences grant P20 GM103650 and National Institute on Aging grant R15 AG052931. We would also like to thank Matthew Bauer and David Knupp for critical review of this chapter.

References

1. Jeck WR, Sorrentino JA, Wang K et al (2013) Circular RNAs are abundant, conserved, and associated with ALU repeats. RNA 19:141–157. https://doi.org/10.1261/rna.035667.112

2. Memczak S, Jens M, Elefsinioti A et al (2013) Circular RNAs are a large class of animal RNAs with regulatory potency. Nature 495:333–338. https://doi.org/10.1038/nature11928

3. Ashwal-Fluss R, Meyer M, Pamudurti NR et al (2014) CircRNA biogenesis competes with pre-mRNA splicing. Mol Cell 56:55–66. https://doi.org/10.1016/j.molcel.2014.08.019

4. Rybak-Wolf A, Stottmeister C, Glazar P et al (2014) Circular RNAs in the mammalian brain are highly abundant, conserved, and dynamically expressed. Mol Cell 58:870–885. https://doi.org/10.1016/j.molcel.2015.03.027

5. Gruner H, Cortés-López M, Cooper DA et al (2016) CircRNA accumulation in the aging mouse brain. Sci Rep 6:38907. https://doi.org/10.1038/srep38907

6. Wang PL, Bao Y, Yee M-C et al (2014) Circular RNA is expressed across the eukaryotic tree of life. PLoS One 9:e90859. https://doi.org/10.1371/journal.pone.0090859

7. Shen Y, Guo X, Wang W (2017) Identification and characterization of circular RNAs in zebrafish. FEBS Lett 591:213–220. https://doi.org/10.1002/1873-3468.12500

8. Westholm JO, Miura P, Olson S et al (2014) Genome-wide analysis of Drosophila circular RNAs reveals their structural and sequence properties and age-dependent neural accumulation. Cell Rep 9:1966–1980. https://doi.org/10.1016/j.celrep.2014.10.062

9. Sun X, Wang L, Ding J et al (2016) Integrative analysis of Arabidopsis thaliana transcriptomics reveals intuitive splicing mechanism for circular RNA. FEBS Lett 590:3510–3516. https://doi.org/10.1002/1873-3468.12440

10. Ye C-Y, Chen L, Liu C et al (2015) Widespread noncoding circular RNAs in plants. New Phytol 208:88–95. https://doi.org/10.1111/nph.13585

11. Nitsche A, Doose G, Tafer H et al (2014) Atypical RNAs in the coelacanth transcriptome. J Exp Zool Part B Mol Dev Evol 322:342–351. https://doi.org/10.1002/jez.b.22542

12. Salzman J, Chen RE, Olsen MN et al (2013) Cell-type specific features of circular RNA expression. PLoS Genet 9:e1003777. https://doi.org/10.1371/journal.pgen.1003777

13. Zhang X-O, Wang H-B, Zhang Y et al (2014) Complementary sequence-mediated exon circularization. Cell 159:134–147. https://doi.org/10.1016/j.cell.2014.09.001

14. Gao Y, Wang J, Zhao F (2015) CIRI: an efficient and unbiased algorithm for de novo circular RNA identification. Genome Biol 16:4. https://doi.org/10.1186/s13059-014-0571-3

15. Szabo L, Morey R, Palpant NJ et al (2015) Statistically based splicing detection reveals neural enrichment and tissue-specific induction of circular RNA during human fetal development. Genome Biol 16:126. https://doi.org/10.1186/s13059-015-0690-5

16. Song X, Zhang N, Han P et al (2016) Circular RNA profile in gliomas revealed by identification tool UROBORUS. Nucleic Acids Res 44:e87. https://doi.org/10.1093/nar/gkw075

17. Zhang Y, Zhang XO, Chen T et al (2013) Circular intronic long noncoding RNAs. Mol Cell 51:792–806. https://doi.org/10.1016/j.molcel.2013.08.017

18. Quinlan AR, Hall IM (2010) BEDTools: a flexible suite of utilities for comparing genomic features. Bioinformatics 26:841–842. https://doi.org/10.1093/bioinformatics/btq033

19. Langmead B, Salzberg SL (2012) Fast gapped-read alignment with Bowtie2. Nat Methods 9:357–360. https://doi.org/10.1038/nmeth.1923

20. Li H, Handsaker B, Wysoker A et al (2009) The sequence alignment/map format and SAMtools. Bioinformatics 25:2078–2079. https://doi.org/10.1093/bioinformatics/btp352

21. Li H (2011) A statistical framework for SNP calling, mutation discovery, association mapping and population genetical parameter estimation from sequencing data. Bioinformatics 27:2987–2993. https://doi.org/10.1093/bioinformatics/btr509

22. Liao Y, Smyth GK, Shi W (2014) FeatureCounts: an efficient general purpose program for assigning sequence reads to genomic features. Bioinformatics 30:923–930. https://doi.org/10.1093/bioinformatics/btt656

23. Thorvaldsdóttir H, Robinson JT, Mesirov JP (2012) Integrative Genomics Viewer (IGV): high-performance genomics data visualization and exploration. Brief Bioinform 14:178–192. https://doi.org/10.1093/bib/bbs017

24. Robinson J, Thorvaldsdóttir H, Winckler W (2011) Integrative genomics viewer. Nat Biotechnol 29:24–26. https://doi.org/10.1038/nbt0111-24

25. Core Team R (2016) R: a language and environment for statistical computing. R Foundation for Statistical Computing, Vienna, Austria. https://www.R-project.org/

26. Wickham H (2009) ggplot2: elegant graphics for data analysis. Springer-Verlag, New York

27. Kivioja T, Vähärautio A, Karlsson K et al (2012) Counting absolute numbers of molecules using unique molecular identifiers. Nat Methods 9:72–74. https://doi.org/10.1038/nmeth.1778

28. Ebbert MTW, Wadsworth ME, Staley LA et al (2016) Evaluating the necessity of PCR duplicate removal from next-generation sequencing data and a comparison of approaches. BMC Bioinformatics 17:239. https://doi.org/10.1186/s12859-016-1097-3

29. Parekh S, Ziegenhain C, Vieth B et al (2016) The impact of amplification on differential expression analyses by RNA-seq. Sci Rep 6:25533. https://doi.org/10.1038/srep25533

30. Martin M (2011) Cutadapt removes adapter sequences from high-throughput sequencing reads. EMBnet J 17:10–12. 10.14806/ej.17.1.200

31. Kent WJ, Sugnet CW, Furey TS et al (2002) the human genome browser at UCSC. Genome Res 12:996–1006. https://doi.org/10.1101/gr.229102

32. Salzman J, Gawad C, Wang PL et al (2012) Circular RNAs are the predominant transcript isoform from hundreds of human genes in diverse cell types. PLoS One 7:e30733. https://doi.org/10.1371/journal.pone.0030733

33. Dou Y, Cha DJ, Franklin JL et al (2016) Circular RNAs are down-regulated in KRAS mutant colon cancer cells and can be transferred to exosomes. Sci Rep 6:37982. https://doi.org/10.1038/srep37982

34. Ivanov A, Memczak S, Wyler E et al (2015) Analysis of intron sequences reveals hallmarks of circular RNA biogenesis in animals. Cell Rep 10:170–177. https://doi.org/10.1016/j.celrep.2014.12.019

35. Glazar P, Papavasileiou P, Rajewsky N (2014) circBase: a database for circular RNAs. RNA 20:1666–1670. https://doi.org/10.1261/rna.043687.113

36. Chen X, Han P, Zhou T et al (2016) circRNADb: a comprehensive database for human circular RNAs with protein-coding annotations. Sci Rep 6:34985. https://doi.org/10.1038/srep34985

37. Liu Y-C, Li J-R, Sun C-H et al (2016) CircNet: a database of circular RNAs derived from transcriptome sequencing data. Nucleic Acids Res 44:D209–D215. https://doi.org/10.1093/nar/gkv940

38. Xia S, Feng J, Lei L et al (2016) Comprehensive characterization of tissue-specific circular RNAs in the human and mouse genomes. Brief Bioinform:1–9. https://doi.org/10.1093/bib/bbw081

Chapter 4

Analysis of Circular RNAs Using the Web Tool CircInteractome

Amaresh C. Panda, Dawood B. Dudekula, Kotb Abdelmohsen, and Myriam Gorospe

Abstract

Circular RNAs (circRNAs) are generated through nonlinear back splicing, during which the 5′ and 3′ ends are covalently joined. Consequently, the lack of free ends makes them very stable compared to their counterpart linear RNAs. By selectively interacting with microRNAs and RNA-binding proteins (RBPs), circRNAs have been shown to influence gene expression programs. We designed a web tool, CircInteractome, in order to (1) explore potential interactions of circRNAs with RBPs, (2) design specific divergent primers to detect circRNAs, (3) study tissue- and cell-specific circRNAs, (4) identify gene-specific circRNAs, (5) explore potential miRNAs interacting with circRNAs, and (6) design specific siRNAs to silence circRNAs. Here, we review the CircInteractome tool and explain recent updates to the site. The database is freely accessible at http://circinteractome.nia.nih.gov.

Key words RNA-binding proteins, Gene-specific circRNAs, Divergent primer design, Cell- and tissue-specific circRNAs, Transcriptome, CLIP-seq

1 Introduction

The past few decades have yielded an ever-growing list of noncoding RNA species with various functions [1]. Circular RNAs (circRNAs) represent a new class of widely expressed and abundant RNA species in eukaryotes [2]. They are generally formed by "head-to-tail" or "back splicing" of pre-mRNA, whereby the 5′ and 3′ ends are covalently linked to form a closed RNA molecule [3, 4]. Although circRNAs have been known for many years, their functions are not as well characterized as those of other noncoding (nc)RNAs such as microRNAs (miRNAs) and long ncRNAs (lncRNAs). However, recent studies have discovered that circRNAs can alter gene expression by interacting with, and in some cases sequestering, miRNAs, RBPs, and splicing factors, thereby altering their availability to protein-coding mRNAs [5, 6]. It has also been suggested that circRNAs could regulate mRNA transcription and translation by interacting

Christoph Dieterich and Argyris Papantonis (eds.), *Circular RNAs: Methods and Protocols*, Methods in Molecular Biology, vol. 1724, https://doi.org/10.1007/978-1-4939-7562-4_4, © Springer Science+Business Media, LLC 2018

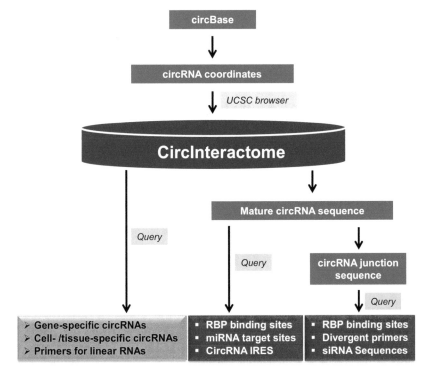

Fig. 1 Workflow of the web tool Circular RNA Interactome or "CircInteractome"

with specific RNAs and proteins [5], and the presence of internal ribosome entry sites (IRESs) on some circRNAs has prompted the suggestion that some circRNAs may be translated [7].

RBPs potently regulate gene expression programs at multiple posttranscriptional levels [8]. Recent developments in the analysis of RNA-protein (RNP) interactions using cross-linking techniques have identified with unprecedented precision the binding sequences of RBPs on target RNAs. MicroRNAs are another major class of factors that control gene expression, generally by associating with target mRNAs that share partial complementarity and suppressing mRNA translation and/or stability [9]. We recently developed a new computational resource named "CircInteractome" [7] which enables the systematic exploration of possible interactions of human circRNAs with RBPs and miRNAs (Fig. 1). In this chapter, we describe in detail this tool and the latest updates we have incorporated into it.

2   Materials

1. Desktop with Windows operating system (Mac OSX and Linux are adequate too) and Internet Explorer, Mozilla Firefox, or Google Chrome browsers.

2. Microsoft Internet Explorer or Mozilla Firefox or Google Chrome browsers.

3 Methods

3.1 Analysis of Interactions of RBPs with circRNAs (Fig. 2)

CircInteractome uses circRNA IDs described in CircBase (http://www.circbase.org), a public database that was developed to gather unified datasets of circRNA IDs, genomic coordinates, and transcripts [10]. The data provided in CircInteractome are predicted based on sequence matches; accordingly, the impact of potential secondary or tertiary structures on circRNA sequence available for interaction with RBPs cannot be considered systematically. Thus, experimental validation is essential to verify circRNA binding to a predicted RBP.

1. Type http://circinteractome.nia.nih.gov into the browser and click "Enter". The home page briefly explains the use of CircInteractome.

2. Click on the "circRNA" tab on the left side.

3. Enter the name of the circRNA (e.g., hsa_circ_0000067) in the specified field and click "circRNA Search".

4. The new page will show the following features for the "hsa_circ_0000067":

    (a) Genomic location

    (b) Length of the genomic and mature circRNA sequences

    (c) Best matched counterpart mRNA (best transcript)

    (d) Tissues or cell lines where this circRNA was detected (Samples)

    (e) Studies reporting this circRNA (Study)

5. This webpage also shows the RBPs with possible binding sites on this circRNA. For instance, hsa_circ_0000067 has five binding sites for AGO2 and two binding sites for HuR (ELAVL1).

6. The user can further search for the RBP-binding sites on the circRNA junction sequence and flanking region. For example, HNRNPC has one site in the flanking sequence upstream of hsa_circ_0000067.

3.2 CircRNA Genomic Sequence and Mature circRNA Sequence (Fig. 3)

It can be challenging to find the mature circRNA sequence from the UCSC browser mirror (http://genome.mdc-berlin.de). With CircInteractome, the user can easily access genomic and mature circRNA sequences following a few simple steps. The circRNAs are usually predicted from unique junction sequences. The sequence of mature circRNA is predicted from the exon sequences present in

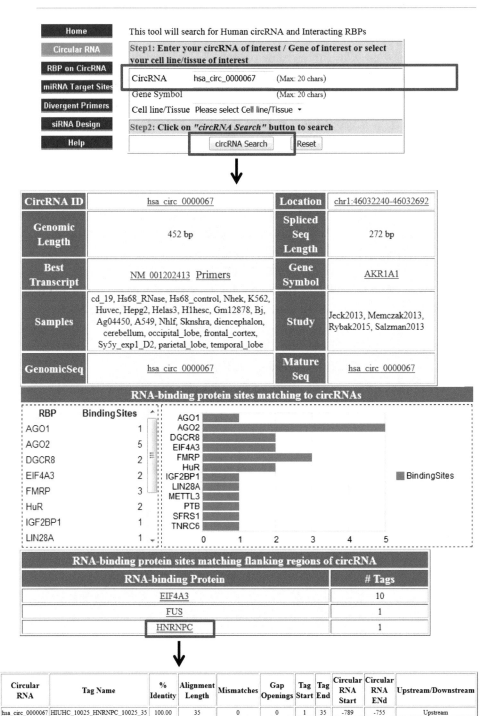

Fig. 2 View of CircInteractome input and output pages. Screenshot of "Circular RNA search" for hsa_circ_0000067, showing RBPs binding to the body and the flanking sequence of this circRNA

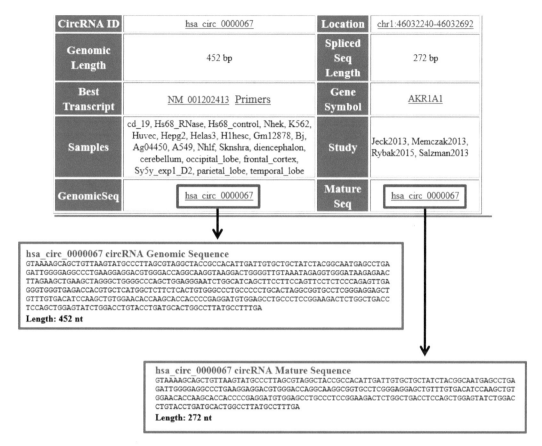

CircRNA ID	hsa_circ_0000067	Location	chr1:46032240-46032692
Genomic Length	452 bp	Spliced Seq Length	272 bp
Best Transcript	NM_001202413 Primers	Gene Symbol	AKR1A1
Samples	cd_19, Hs68_RNase, Hs68_control, Nhek, K562, Huvec, Hepg2, Helas3, H1hesc, Gm12878, Bj, Ag04450, A549, Nhlf, Sknshra, diencephalon, cerebellum, occipital_lobe, frontal_cortex, Sy5y_exp1_D2, parietal_lobe, temporal_lobe	Study	Jeck2013, Memczak2013, Rybak2015, Salzman2013
GenomicSeq	hsa_circ_0000067	Mature Seq	hsa_circ_0000067

hsa_circ_0000067 circRNA Genomic Sequence
GTAAAAGCAGCTGTTAAGTATGCCCTTAGCGTAGGCTACCGCCACATTGATTGTGCTGCTATCTACGGCAATGAGCCTGA
GATTGGGGAGGCCCTGAAGGAGGACGTGGGACCAGGCAAGGTAAGGACTGGGGTTGTAAATAGAGGTGGGATAAGAGAAC
TTAGAAGCTGAAGCTAGGGCTGGGGCCCAGCTGGAGGGAATCTGGCATCAGCTTCCTTCCAGTTCCTCTCCCAGAGTTGA
GGGTGGGTGAGACCACGTGCTCATGGCTCTTCTCACTGTGGGCCCTGCCCCCTGCACTAGGCGGTGCCTCGGGAGGAGCT
GTTTGTGACATCCAAGCTGTGGAACACCAAGCACCACCCCGAGGATGTGGAGCCTGCCCTCCGGAAGACTCTGGCTGACC
TCCAGCTGGAGTATCTGGACCTGTACCTGATGCACTGGCCTTATGCCTTTGA
Length: 452 nt

hsa_circ_0000067 circRNA Mature Sequence
GTAAAAGCAGCTGTTAAGTATGCCCTTAGCGTAGGCTACCGCCACATTGATTGTGCTGCTATCTACGGCAATGAGCCTGA
GATTGGGGAGGCCCTGAAGGAGGACGTGGGACCAGGCAAGGCGGTGCCTCGGGAGGAGCTGTTTGTGACATCCAAGCTGT
GGAACACCAAGCACCACCCCGAGGATGTGGAGCCTGCCCTCCGGAAGACTCTGGCTGACCTCCAGCTGGAGTATCTGGAC
CTGTACCTGATGCACTGGCCTTATGCCTTTGA
Length: 272 nt

Fig. 3 Genomic and mature sequences of a given circRNA. Illustrative screenshots from the CircInteractome showing the genomic (left) and mature circRNA (right) sequence for hsa_ circ_0000067

that specific genomic location. Further multi-exon circRNAs may or may not include all of the exons and introns in the mature circRNA forms, which will need to be verified experimentally.

1. Type http://circinteractome.nia.nih.gov in the web browser and click "Enter".
2. Click on the "Circular RNA" tab on the left side.
3. Enter the name of the circRNA (e.g., hsa_circ_0000067) in the specified field and click on the "circRNA Search".
4. The new webpage shows various features for the "hsa_circ_0000067".
5. Click on the "hsa_circ_0000067" next to "GenomicSeq" or "Mature Seq" to find the genomic or mature circRNA sequence, respectively.

3.3 Specific circRNA Gene (Fig. 4)

1. Type http://circinteractome.nia.nih.gov in the web browser and click "Enter".

2. Click on the "Circular RNA" tab on the left side.

3. Enter the name of the gene, e.g., *GAPDH*, on the specified field and click on the "circRNA Search".

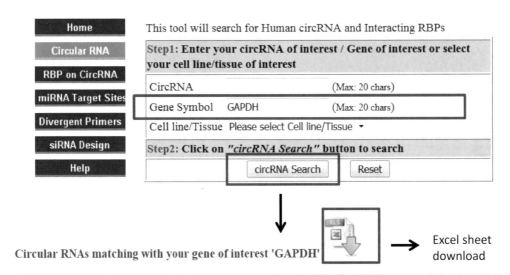

Fig. 4 Gene-specific circRNAs. For a given gene symbol entered, the circRNAs generated from that gene are identified

4. The new page shows a table containing the name, genomic location, and length of circRNAs generated from the *GAPDH* gene.

5. This table also includes the tissues and cell types wherein the circRNAs were detected (below).

6. The user can also download the table as an Excel spreadsheet by clicking on the "excel sheet" logo on top of the table.

3.4 Cell Types and Tissues Where circRNAs Are Expressed (Fig. 5)

1. Type http://circinteractome.nia.nih.gov in the web browser and click "Enter".

2. Click on the "Circular RNA" tab on the left side.

3. Select the name of the tissue or cell type of interest (e.g., HEK293) from the drag-down list and click on the "circRNA Search".

4. The new page shows a table containing the name, genomic location, and length of circRNAs expressed in HEK293 cells.

5. This table also shows other tissues or cell types where these circRNAs are reported to be expressed along with HEK293 cells (highlighted).

6. The user can also download the table in the form of Excel spreadsheet by clicking on the "excel sheet" logo on top of the table.

3.5 miRNAs Targeting circRNAs (Fig. 6)

Note: The predicted miRNAs may not bind to circRNAs in vivo due to a lack of accessibility of binding site or lack of miRNA expression. As for RBPs, experimental validation is also necessary for microRNAs. Furthermore, miRNAs which interact in vivo but are not predicted by TargetScan search algorithms may be missed.

1. Type http://circinteractome.nia.nih.gov into the browser and click "Enter".

2. Click on the "miRNA Target Sites" tab on the left side.

3. Enter the name of the circRNA (e.g., hsa_circ_0000094) in the specified field and click on the "miRNA Target Search". CircInteractome uses the TargetScan Perl script to predict the miRNAs which have sequence complementarity with circRNAs [11].

4. The new page shows the predicted miRNAs and number of sites in "hsa_circ_0000094".

5. This page also shows base-pairing and details of the miRNA-circRNA interactions.

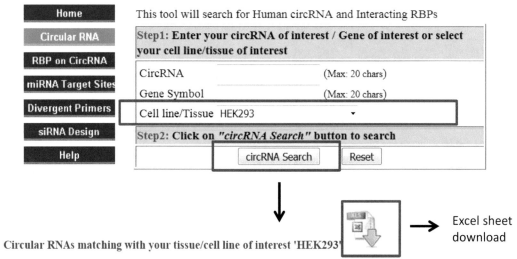

Fig. 5 Cell/tissue-specific circRNAs. CircRNAs identified in previous studies in specific cell types or tissues are identified

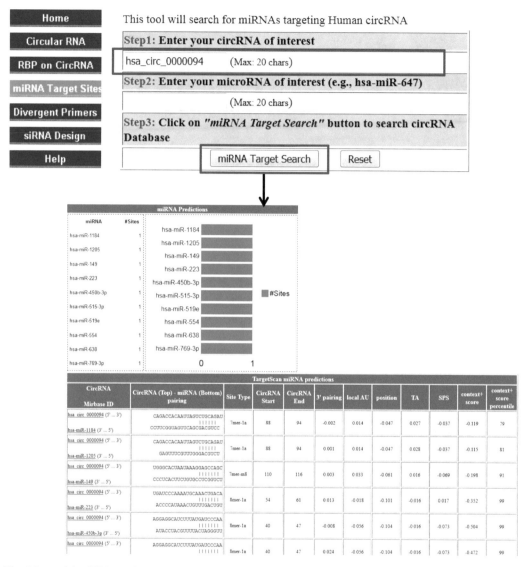

Fig. 6 Potential miRNA-circRNA interactions. For a given circRNA ID entered (hsa_circ_0000094), the miRNAs potentially targeting hsa_circ_0000094 are identified

3.6 CircRNA Divergent Primer Design (Fig. 7)

Note: The divergent primers designed here may detect the circRNA splice variants coming from the same primary transcript. The user may need to sequence the PCR product to find the exact circRNA junction of interest.

1. Type http://circinteractome.nia.nih.gov in the web browser and click "Enter".

2. Click on the "Divergent Primers" tab on the left side.

3. Enter the name of the circRNA (e.g., hsa_circ_0000094) in the specified field and click on the "Divergent Primers Search".

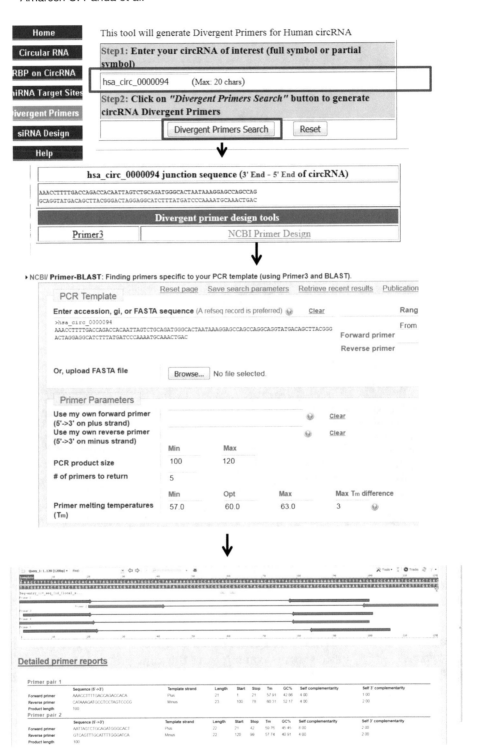

Fig. 7 Divergent primer design. Screenshots of input and output webpage for divergent primer design for hsa_circ_0000094. Screenshot of the output page showing the junction sequence of circRNA and links of primer design tools (Primer3 and NCBI)

4. The new page shows the circRNA junction sequence and two options for divergent primer design.

5. The user can click on either "Primer3" or "NCBI Primer Design" and the new webpage will design five pairs of primers for the circRNA of interest "hsa_circ_0000094".

3.7 Designing Primers for Linear Counterpart RNA (Fig. 8)

1. Type http://circinteractome.nia.nih.gov in the web browser and click "Enter".

2. Click on the "Circular RNA" tab on the left side.

3. Enter the name of the circRNA (e.g., hsa_circ_0000094) on the specified field and click on the "circRNA Search".

4. The new page shows the following features for the "hsa_circ_0000094", e.g., genomic location, length of genomic and mature circRNA sequence, and best matching counterpart mRNA (best transcript).

5. Clicking the hyperlink "Primers" next to "Best Transcript" will open a new page for NCBI primer design tool. The user can design primers by clicking on the "Primers" tab.

3.8 siRNAs Targeting circRNAs (Fig. 9)

Note: The siRNAs have at least ten nucleotides base pairing with the linear counterpart mRNA which might work as miRNA/siRNA. The user may try several siRNAs to identify one that specifically knocks down the circRNA without affecting the linear counterpart mRNA.

1. Type http://circinteractome.nia.nih.gov in the browser and click "Enter".

2. Click on the "siRNA Design" tab on the left side.

3. Enter the name of the circRNA, e.g., hsa_circ_0000094, in the specified field and click on the "siRNA Search".

4. The new webpage shows the ten best possible siRNA target sequences for "hsa_circ_0000094".

5. The users may purchase the siRNAs from any source. However, links to order siRNAs from IDT or Dharmacon are provided. The user may wish to add two additional nucleotides (dTdT) as 3′ DNA overhangs to the siRNA for better silencing effects.

4 Summary

1. In summary, CircInteractome facilitates the study of circRNAs, as well as the RBPs and nucleic acids with which circRNAs associate. The information provided by this tool can illuminate possible functions of circRNAs as molecules that (1) sequester RBPs, microRNAs, and/or other interacting molecules to reduce their availability to mRNAs, (2) function as potential support structures

CircRNA ID	hsa_circ_0000094	Location	chr1:95364926-95365046
Genomic Length	120 bp	Spliced Seq Length	120 bp
Best Transcript	NM_001839 Primers	Gene Symbol	CNN3
Samples	HEK293, Sy5y_exp_D2	Study	Memczak2013, Rybak2015
GenomicSeq	hsa_circ_0000094	Mature Seq	hsa_circ_0000094

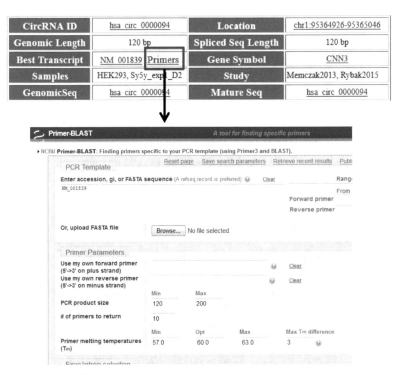

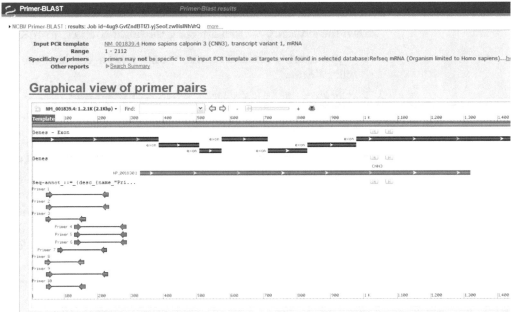

Fig. 8 Primer design for counterpart linear RNA. Screenshots of input and output webpage for designing primer for the linear RNA counterpart using NCBI primer design tool

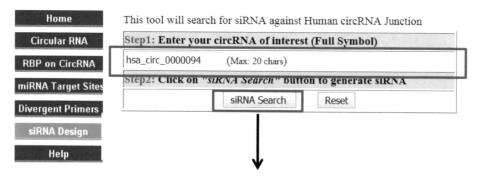

Fig. 9 CircRNA siRNA design. Screenshot of input and output webpage of CircInteractome siRNA design, including an example of output siRNAs targeting the junction sequence of hsa_ circ_0000094

for the assembly of multimolecular complexes, (3) may be translated giving rise to peptides and proteins, (4) interact with mRNAs, thereby promoting or repressing their stability or translation, etc.

2. CircInteractome facilitates the design of siRNAs for silencing circRNAs and oligomers for detecting (by RT-qPCR analysis) the circRNAs and the parent RNAs from which they arise.

3. CircInteractome will continue to expand to include additional circRNAs, including circRNAs from other species. It will also search against more databases of RBPs, microRNAs, and interacting molecules as they become available.

4. Collectively, CircInteractome will accelerate our efforts to elucidate the functions of circRNAs in development and disease.

Acknowledgments

This work was supported in full by the National Institute on Aging Intramural Research Program, National Institutes of Health.

References

1. Morris KV, Mattick JS (2014) The rise of regulatory RNA. Nat Rev Genet 15:423–437

2. Jeck WR, Sorrentino JA, Wang K, Slevin MK, Burd CE, Liu J, Marzluff WF, Sharpless NE (2013) Circular RNAs are abundant, conserved, and associated with ALU repeats. RNA 19:141–157

3. Schindewolf C, Braun S, Domdey H (1996) In vitro generation of a circular exon from a linear pre-mRNA transcript. Nucleic Acids Res 24:1260–1266

4. Starke S, Jost I, Rossbach O, Schneider T, Schreiner S, Hung LH, Bindereif A (2015) Exon circularization requires canonical splice signals. Cell Rep 10:103–111

5. Chen LL (2016) The biogenesis and emerging roles of circular RNAs. Nat Rev Mol Cell Biol 17:205–211

6. Hansen TB, Jensen TI, Clausen BH, Bramsen JB, Finsen B, Damgaard CK, Kjems J (2013) Natural RNA circles function as efficient microRNA sponges. Nature 495:384–388

7. Dudekula DB, Panda AC, Grammatikakis I, De S, Abdelmohsen K, Gorospe M (2016) CircInteractome: a web tool for exploring circular RNAs and their interacting proteins and microRNAs. RNA Biol 13:34–42

8. Glisovic T, Bachorik JL, Yong J, Dreyfuss G (2008) RNA-binding proteins and post-transcriptional gene regulation. FEBS Lett 582:1977–1986

9. Behm-Ansmant I, Rehwinkel J, Izaurralde E (2006) MicroRNAs silence gene expression by repressing protein expression and/or by promoting mRNA decay. Cold Spring Harb Symp Quant Biol 71:523–530

10. Glazar P, Papavasileiou P, Rajewsky N (2014) circBase: a database for circular RNAs. RNA 20:1666–1670

11. Grimson A, Farh KK, Johnston WK, Garrett-Engele P, Lim LP, Bartel DP (2007) MicroRNA targeting specificity in mammals: determinants beyond seed pairing. Mol Cell 27:91–105

Chapter 5

Characterization and Validation of Circular RNA and Their Host Gene mRNA Expression Using PCR

Andreas W. Heumüller and Jes-Niels Boeckel

Abstract

Polymerase chain reaction enables the detection and characterization of circular RNA expression. The use of divergent primer pairs flanking the back-splice site, being the unique sequence element of a circular RNA, enables the detection of circular RNA expression. Here we describe the basic techniques to detect different circular transcripts of a gene or one circular RNA specifically by PCR and highlight the advantages and drawbacks of both.

Key words Divergent primer, Circular RNA, Polymerase chain reaction, Back-splice site, CircRNA

1 Introduction

Detection of circular RNA (circRNA) expression can be achieved using polymerase chain reaction (PCR) [1], northern blot [1], 2D gel electrophoresis [2], gel trap electrophoresis [1, 3], in situ hybridization [4], and RNase H degradation assay [5, 6]. PCR is currently the fastest and easiest method to detect the expression of circular RNAs. Primers used in PCR for detection of protein-coding or noncoding RNAs are necessarily designed in a convergent direction to allow amplification of the primer-flanked nucleic acid region. For detection of circRNA expression using PCR, however, the use of divergent orientated primer pairs is necessary [1]. Here we demonstrate the basic techniques to detect different circular transcripts or one circular RNA of a gene by semiquantitative and quantitative PCR, and the subsequent purification of the PCR product for validation of the back-splice site using Sanger sequencing. Back-splice sequence information of circular transcripts can be obtained by RNA-sequencing data [7–9] or publicly accessible sets of non-poly-A-selected RNA-sequencing data in the NCBI GEO database (ncbi.nlm.nih.gov/geo). Primers to specifically detect circRNAs by PCR should be designed divergently which can be easily achieved using free online tools such as primer3 (primer3.ut.ee)

Christoph Dieterich and Argyris Papantonis (eds.), *Circular RNAs: Methods and Protocols*, Methods in Molecular Biology, vol. 1724, https://doi.org/10.1007/978-1-4939-7562-4_5, © Springer Science+Business Media, LLC 2018

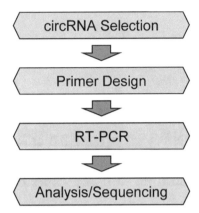

Fig. 1 Workflow for circRNA analysis. Selection of circRNAs from database, microarray, or next-generation sequencing is followed by primer design. Next, semi- and/or quantitative polymerase chain reaction with divergent primer pairs is used to validate the expression of the selected candidate circRNA. For final validation and control, Sanger sequencing of the obtained PCR product is recommended

[10, 11]. Amplification of circRNA transcripts for the first time using semiquantitative PCR and subsequent analysis by gel electrophoresis is recommended since one host gene can give rise to several circRNA splice variants with the same or even varying back-splice sites [12]. Furthermore, quantitative PCR enables the fast and high-throughput analysis of circRNA expression levels. Specificity of qPCR results can be analyzed by the melting curve of the qPCR product and processing of a negative control, e.g., -RT or H_2O control. However, amplification of the back-splice site-specific sequence should at least once be validated by Sanger sequencing, especially when analyzing a yet-not-validated or characterized circRNA (*see* Fig. 1).

2 Materials and Tools

Prepare all solutions using DNase- and RNase-free water. Wear gloves at all times to avoid sample contamination with RNases or genomic DNA. Diligently follow waste disposal regulation when disposing waste material.

2.1 Primer Design

1. CircRNA-Sequencing data with back-splice site location and sequence information.

2. Web tool for primer design such as http://primer3.ut.ee.

3. Web tool for in silico PCR such as https://genome.ucsc.edu/cgi-bin/hgPcr.

2.2 Semiquantitative PCR (The Use of Taq Polymerase Is Shown as an Example (See Note 1))

1. Random hexamer-primed cDNA (5 ng/μL) (*see* **Note 2**) *Taq* polymerase (Hot-start) (*see* **Note 1**) *Taq* reaction buffer (10×): —500 mM KCl—15 mM $MgCl_2$—pH 8.3 at 25 °C.

2. 10 mM dNTPs (dATP, dCTP, dGTP, dTTP).

3. Primer stocks 10 μM each.

4. DNase/RNase-free water.

5. Reaction tubes.

6. PCR thermal cycler.

2.3 Quantitative PCR

1. Random hexamer-primed cDNA (5 ng/μL) (*see* **Note 2**).

2. 96-Well plates (or PCR stripes or single-PCR tubes).

3. Adhesive covering films (in case PCR plates are used).

4. SYBR Green Master Mix:

   (a) 10–20 mM Tris—HCl (concentration can be optimized)

   (b) 50–100 mM KCl (concentration can be optimized)

   (c) 3–6 mM $MgCl_2$ (concentration can be optimized)

   (d) 0.2–0.4 mM dNTPs (dATP, dCTP, dGTP, dTTP) (concentration can be optimized)

   (e) *Taq* polymerase (Hot-start) (*see* **Note 1**)

   (f) Internal reference dye (1×), e.g., ROX (Optional! In case PCR thermal cycler supplier recommends the use)

   (g) PCR stabilizers (optional)

   (h) SYBR Green Dye

5. DNase/RNase-free water.

6. Primer stocks 10 μM each.

7. PCR thermal cycler.

2.4 Purification of the PCR Product for Sanger Sequencing

1. Phenol/chloroform/isoamyl alcohol (25:24:1(v/v/v)).

2. Cold ethanol.

3. TE-Buffer.

4. Centrifuge for 1.5 mL tubes.

5. Heat block for 1.5 mL tubes.

6. Primer stocks 10 μM each.

3 Method

3.1 Primer Design

1. Determine the chromosome location of the ends predicted to pair during back splicing in your sequencing dataset (or directly extract the back-splice reads from the RNA-seq data, go to **step 5**) (*see* **Note 3**). Determine which exons/introns are

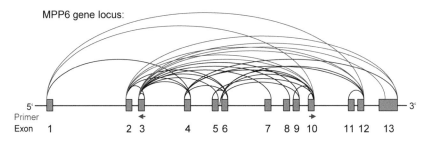

Fig. 2 RNA splicing scheme of the human MPP6 gene locus. Exons of the human MPP6 gene are depicted in grey. Potential back-splicing combinations forming circRNAs annotated in the circbase databank are implied by semicircles. Red semicircles refer to those circRNAs which are in principle detectable with the divergent primer pair (red arrows)

included in the back splicing using the genome browser and the chromosomal locations (to get an easy overview of the involved exons in your circRNA, insert the whole back-splice site sequence in the "blat" tool under tools at https://genome.ucsc.edu/cgi-bin/hgPcr) (*see* Fig. 2a).

2. Fetch the corresponding exon sequence to your respective gene and species from www.ensembl.org (*see* Fig. 3a).

3. Reverse the exon order (paste the sequence of the latter exon in front of the prior), but keep the 5′→3′ orientation of both exons (*see* Fig. 3a, b).

4. Paste the sequence into the corresponding box at http://primer3.ut.ee/.

5. Change box "Product-size range" to 70–150 bp and choose pick primers (size of 40–120 bp is often recommended by qPCR thermal cycler suppliers; for semiquantitative PCR also bigger product sizes can be chosen) (*see* Fig. 3b).

6. Choose primer pair, ensure that the amplified region covers the back-splice site, and check that predicted primer T_M is close to 60 °C. Both primers should not overlap the back-splice site (*see* **Note 4**).

7. Paste primer sequence in the UCSC in silico PCR tool and check amplification in the genome assembly and the UCSC annotated genes; no predicted amplification is expected (*see* **Note 5**)!

3.2 PCR
Semiquantitative PCR

The following protocol is described for the amplification of circular RNAs. For reference, expression of the linear RNA of the gene of interest should be assessed additionally (*see* **Note 6**).

1. Thaw buffer concentrate, dNTP mix, and random hexamer-primed cDNA on ice (*see* **Note 2**).

A

Exon 3 (ENSE00000831999):

5'agcagCAATGCAGCAAGTCTTGGAAAACCTTACGGAGCTGCCCTCGTCTACTGGAGCAGAAGA
AATAGACCTAATTTTCCTCAAGGGAATTATGGAGAATCCTATTGTAAAATCACTTGCTAAGgtata3'

....

Exons 4-9

....

Exon 10 (ENSE00003556537):

5'tttagAATTTGATCGTCATGAAATCCAGATATATGAGGAGGTAGCCAAAATGCCTCCCTTCCAGA
GAAAAACATTAGTATTGATAGGAGCTCAAGGTGTAGGCCGAAGAAGCTTGAAAAACAGGTTCAT
AGTATTGAATCCCACTAGATTTGGAACTACGGTGCCATgtaag3'

B

Expected backsplice-site for hsa_circ_0133996 (circMPP6):

5'-Exon10-3'→5'-Exon 3-3'

5'AATTTGATCGTCATGAAATCCAGATATATGAGGAGGTAGCCAAAATGCCTCCCTTCCAGAGAA

AAACATTAGTATTGATAGGAGCTCAAGGTGTAGGCCGAAGAAGCTTGAAAAACAGGTTCATAG

TATTGAATCCCACTAGATTTGGAACTACGGTGCCAT**3'**   **5'CAATGCAGCAAGTCTTGGAAAAC**

CTTACGGAGCTGCCCTCGTCTACTGGAGCAGAAGAAATAGACCTAATTTTCCTCAAGGGAATTA

TGGAGAATCCTATTGTAAAATCACTTGCTAAG**3'**

Fig. 3 Primer design for the circRNA hsa_circ_0133996 (circMPP6). (**a**) DNA sequence of the exon 3 (ENSE00000831999) and exon 10 (ENSE00003556537) taken from ensembl.org (HG38). Intronic sequences are shown in lowercase and light grey. (**b**) Scrambling the exon order generates the potential back-splice site (BSS; yellow). CircRNA detection by PCR is enabled using divergent primer pairs, which are in convergent direction following back splicing. Primer locations and directions are indicated in red resulting in a predicted PCR product size of 95 bp for hsa_circ_0133996

2. Calculate the number of reactions and include 1–2 additional reactions to compensate for eventual loss by pipetting. Prepare PCR master mix as follows:

   (a) *Taq* reaction buffer (10×)   2.5 μL
   (b) 10 mM dNTPs   0.5 μL
   (c) *Taq* polymerase (1 U/μL)   1 μL
   (d) Forward primer   1 μL
   (e) Reverse primer   1 μL
   (f) RNase/DNase-free water   14 μL

3. Distribute 20 μL PCR master mix for each reaction, and add 5 μL random hexamer-primed cDNA (a RNA/cDNA equivalent of >10 ng per reaction is recommended) (*see* **Note 2**). Include a H$_2$O control consisting of 15 μL of the PCR master mix and add 5 μL H$_2$O (*see* **Note 7**).

4. Run PCR using the following protocol:

   (a) 95 °C 2 min

   (b) 95 °C 10 s |

   (c) 60 °C 20 s | ×30–35 PCR cycles

   (d) 72 °C 15 s |

   (e) 4 °C   hold

Note: The temperature and time given in (d) are highly dependent on the respective polymerase and the product size. When using *Taq* polymerase, a suitable temperature of 72 °C should be used in **step 4d** (*see* **Notes 1** and **13**).

5. Analyze PCR products by gel electrophoresis using 2% agarose gels (*see* **Notes 8** and **9**).

3.3 Quantitative PCR

The following protocol is described using the SYBR Green Master Mix for a standard 96-well qPCR. We recommend testing the specificity of the PCR assay for circRNA detection using semi-quantitative PCR and gel electrophoresis prior to qPCR (*see* **Note 13**). Furthermore, the qPCR product should always be processed by melt curve analysis and at least once by subsequent gel electrophoresis (*see* **Note 10**). Melt curve analysis is not necessary, when using hydrolysis probe-based qPCR. In this case, use a hydrolysis probe master mix (which does not contain the SYBR Green Dye but a suitable background dye) instead of the SYBR Green Master Mix in the following protocol (*see* **Note 11**).

1. Thaw SYBR Green Master Mix, primer, and random hexamer-primed cDNA on ice (*see* **Note 2**).

2. Calculate the number of reactions and include 1–2 additional reactions to compensate for eventual loss by pipetting. Prepare qPCR Master Mix (10 μL SYBR Green Master Mix, 3 μL water, 1 μL of the forward and reverse 10 μM primer stock each). When performing hydrolysis probe-based qPCR use 10 μL hydrolysis probe master mix, 2 μL water, 1 μL of the forward and reverse 10 μM primer stock each, and 1 μL of the hydrolysis probe).

3. Distribute 15 μL of the PCR master mix for each reaction, and add 5 μL random hexamer-primed cDNA (*see* **Note 2**). Include a H_2O control consisting of 15 μL of the PCR master mix and add 5 μL H_2O (*see* **Note 3**).

4. Run qPCR using the following protocol:

   (a) 95 °C 20 s

   (b) 95 °C 3 s |

   (c) 60 °C 30 s | ×40

   (d) 95 °C 15 s

(e) 60 °C 60 s

Melt curve analysis (raise 0.05 C/s)

(f) 95 °C 15 s

5. Confirm melt curve for each primer (*see* **Note 12**).

6. Analyze data using the 2^{-CT} method or the $2^{-\Delta CT}$ method when a housekeeping gene (e.g., the mRNA of RPLP0) has been measured.

3.4 Analyzing the PCR Product

PCR products amplifying the back-splice region should be purified using phenol/chloroform/isoamyl alcohol precipitation [13], and subsequently used for Sanger sequencing (PCR sequencing) to validate the existence of the back-splice site and to control the specificity of the divergent-orientated primers used in the PCR.

1. Add an equal volume of phenol/chloroform/isoamyl alcohol (25:24:1 (v/v/v)) to the PCR product in a 1.5 mL reaction tube and mix by vortexing.

2. Centrifuge for 5 min at $12,000 \times g$ at room temperature.

3. Handle the tube carefully, and avoid disturbing the phase separation—transfer the upper (aqueous) phase to a new 1.5 mL reaction tube. Don't disturb the lower (organic) phase; contamination with the lower phase can result in reduced extraction efficiency! Discard the tube containing the lower phase (phenol waste).

4. Mix the sample with 2.5 volumes of cold ethanol and centrifuge for 15 min at maximal speed at 4 °C to precipitate the DNA.

5. Remove as much supernatant as possible with a pipette.

6. The pellet should dry on a heat block with open lid at 37 °C for 0.5–2 min.

7. Resuspend pellet in 10 μL TE buffer.

8. DNA amount should be determined and sample sent to PCR sequencing using the divergent forward and reverse primer.

4 Notes

1. In this protocol the use of *Taq* polymerase is shown as an example; the whole procedure could also be done with other polymerases such as *Kod* or else, which may require different buffer condition.

2. CircRNAs lack polyadenylation. Any RNA reverse transcribed using oligo-dT primers will most likely not allow the detection of circRNAs by PCR. Instead, copy DNA should be transcribed using random hexamer primers.

3. Published sequencing data can yield a fast overview over potential circRNA transcripts (*see* Subheading 3.1). We highly recommend assessing the potential circRNAs resulting from the gene of choice (http://www.circbase.org), prior to primer design to determine which circRNAs in principle can be detected by a respective primer pair and which may not. In general, circRNAs whose paired ends locate upstream of the 5′ located primer and downstream of 3′ located primer can be potentially amplified by the respective primer pair (*see* also Fig. 2a).

4. It is possible to place a primer directly on the back-splice site which allows the specific detection of only one circRNA transcript. However, we do not recommend this strategy, since the properties of the primers (T_M, hairpin structure) are prone to fail good quality standards. Most importantly, such a primer may additionally bind the linear sequence resulting in a PCR product which cannot be distinguished in length from the circRNA PCR product (*see* **step 6** in Subheading 3.1).

5. Due to the lack of algorithms enabling the prediction of scrambled exon PCRs, it is only possible to exclude linear PCR products using in silico PCR prediction tools. Hereby, a specific primer pair for circRNA detection does not yield any predicted PCR products.

6. The regulation of a host gene is very likely contributing to the expressional regulation of all circRNAs this gene gives rise to. Therefore, when analyzing the regulation of a circRNA it is mandatory to also analyze the expression of the respective host gene. Here, primer pairs for analysis of the host gene expression should be positioned apart of the exons forming the respective circRNA (*see* Fig. 6a).

7. Given the low expression levels of many circRNAs [14], negative controls (namely RT and water controls) are to be included. Amplification levels of valid circRNAs should be clearly distinguishable from the negative controls. Since primers are designed in a divergent fashion, linear amplification of non-circRNA transcripts can occur. To exclude such products (*see* [8]), additional controls can include samples amplified with only the forward or the reverse primer (*see* Fig. 4a).

8. Some genes harbor multiple circRNAs and a primer pair flanking one potential back-splice site may therefore detect more than one circular RNA transcript. Bands can be attributed to different circRNAs by evaluating the predicted product size (*see* Fig. 4a, b). Prediction is based on the assumption that only exonic sequences are included in the circRNAs, which is true for the most circRNAs but not all. To determine the product size, first identify those circRNAs whose back-splice site locates

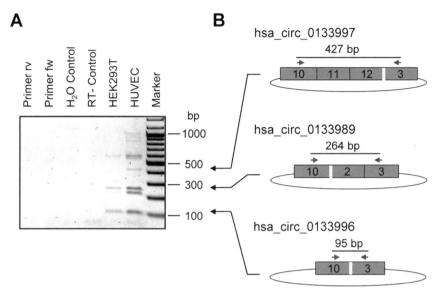

Fig. 4 Validation of circRNA expression using PCR. (**a**) Agarose gel electrophoresis of the PCR products produced by the primer pair shown in Fig. 2. No products are detectable in both the RT and H_2O control. Single-primer controls do not show visible bands, indicating no linear amplification. Amplification using HEK293T and HUVEC cDNA leads to multiple PCR products which are differentially expressed between both cell lines (*see* **Note 13**). (**b**) Schematic display of three different circRNAs produced from the MPP6 gene locus (back-splice site in yellow). The same primer pair (red arrows) enables the detection of all circRNAs. Product size is calculated using the exonic sequences and can be associated with specific bands

to downstream of the forward and upstream of the reverse primer. Subsequently, infer the length of the corresponding exons and sum up the nucleotide count of all exons between the primers and the back-splice site (*see* Fig. 2a). However, definite ascription can only be achieved by Sanger sequencing of the PCR products (*see* Subheading 3.2, **step 3**).

9. We highly recommend to at least once validate the back-splice site of chosen circRNAs by sequencing (*see* Subheading 3.2, **step 3**).

10. Detection of the product of an unknown PCR should be performed for the first time by semiquantitative PCR with subsequent gel electrophoresis and characterization of the PCR product (*see* Figs. 4a, b and 5a, b). The obtained PCR product should be compared to non-template controls such as -RT or H_2O control PCR reactions (*see* Figs. 4a and 5b). Thereafter, the respective circRNA could be analyzed in greater reaction numbers in a qPCR.

11. Hydrolysis probe-based qPCR can be used to increase the specificity of the qPCR reaction and to reduce amplification of multiple circRNAs using a divergent-orientated primer pair (*see* Fig. 4a, b). The primers should be designed as described in

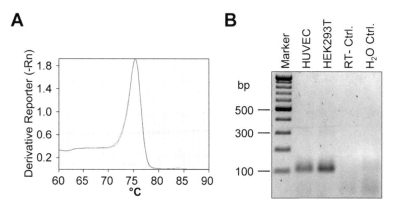

Fig. 5 Validation of circRNA expression using qPCR. (**a**) Melt curve analysis of the products of the divergent primer pair shown in Figs. 3 and 4 (*see* **Note 6**). Graph shows a single peak, referring to a single product from HEK293 (red curve) and HUVEC (blue curve) cDNA. (**b**) Gel electrophoresis analyzing the qPCR product of the PCR reaction shown in Fig. 4a. A single-PCR product, in both HUVEC and HEK293T samples are detected, which is likely resulting only from hsa_circ_0133996 based on the observed bp size. Other larger circRNAs (*see* Fig. 3) are not visible; reduced amplification time in qPCR compared to semiquantitative PCR enables detection of only hsa_circ_0133996 (*see* **Note 13**)

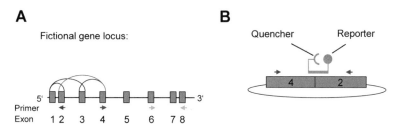

Fig. 6 Specific detection of host genes and circRNAs. (**a**) Scheme of a fictional gene locus showing potential circRNA back splicing. The divergent primer pair (red arrows) enables the detection of one circRNA. The convergent primer pair (blue arrows) allows the detection of exons of the linear host gene, which are not part of any proposed circRNA. Primer for measuring host gene expression should not include exons used for circRNA back splicing or backbone. (**b**) Specific circRNA detection can be achieved using a fluorescent reporter probe overlapping the back-splice site. During amplification, bound probes are digested due to the 5′ ->3′ exonuclease activity of the *Taq* polymerase and reporter and quencher are separated enabling the detection of a fluorescence signal

Subheading 3.1. The hydrolysis probe should have a length of 20–30 bp and should be placed directly on the back-splice site in equal parts on both exons forming the back-splice site (*see* Fig. 6b). This design enables specific detection of only one back-splice site, excluding inclusion of further exons in the PCR product (*see* Fig. 4a, b).

12. When analyzing circRNAs by qPCR, melt curve analysis following the amplification steps should always be included (*see* Fig. 5a). Due to the complexity of the circRNA splicing of a host gene, it is possible that primers amplify more than one circRNA encoded by that host gene. Primer pairs which lead to more than one distinct peak in melt curve analysis should not be used for the quantitative evaluation of circRNA expression levels (*see* Figs. 2a and 4a).

13. Duration of the extension time step in PCR amplification is crucial for specific detection of one circular RNA or more circRNAs from the same host gene. The extension time of 15 s (*see* Subheading 3.2, **step 4**) used in semiquantitative PCR gives rise to several PCR products with varying sizes (*see* Fig. 4a, b). The reduction of the extension time as used in the two-step qPCR method (*see* Subheading 3.3, **step 4c, d**) results in reduction of larger product number synthesis (*see* Fig. 5a, b). Thereby, generation of smaller qPCR products is favoured, which enables more specific detection of the target circRNA expression.

Acknowledgments

This work was supported by the German Cardiac Society (Deutsche Gesellschaft für Kardiologie (DGK)) to Jes-Niels Boeckel.

References

1. Hansen TB, Wiklund ED, Bramsen JB et al (2011) miRNA-dependent gene silencing involving Ago2-mediated cleavage of a circular antisense RNA. EMBO J 30:4414–4422

2. Tabak HF, Van der Horst G, Smit J et al (1988) Discrimination between RNA circles, interlocked RNA circles and lariats using two-dimensional polyacrylamide gel electrophoresis. Nucleic Acids Res 16:6597–6605

3. Schindler CW, Krolewski JJ, Rush MG (1982) Selective trapping of circular double-stranded DNA molecules in solidifying agarose. Plasmid 7:263–270

4. You X, Vlatkovic I, Babic A et al (2015) Neural circular RNAs are derived from synaptic genes and regulated by development and plasticity. Nat Neurosci 18:603–610

5. Capel B, Swain A, Nicolis S et al (1993) Circular transcripts of the testis-determining gene Sry in adult mouse testis. Cell 73:1019–1030

6. Jeck WR, Sharpless NE (2014) Detecting and characterizing circular RNAs. Nat Biotechnol 32:453–461

7. Jeck WR, Sorrentino JA, Wang K et al (2013) Circular RNAs are abundant, conserved, and associated with ALU repeats. RNA 19:141–157

8. Memczak S, Jens M, Elefsinioti A et al (2013) Circular RNAs are a large class of animal RNAs with regulatory potency. Nature 495:333–338

9. Boeckel JN, Jaé N, Heumüller AW et al (2015) Identification and characterization of hypoxia-regulated endothelial circular RNA. Circ Res 117:884–890

10. Untergasser A, Cutcutache I, Koressaar T et al (2012) Primer3—new capabilities and interfaces. Nucleic Acids Res 40:e115

11. Koressaar T, Remm M (2007) Enhancements and modifications of primer design program Primer3. Bioinformatics 23:1289–1291

12. Nigro JM, Cho KR, Fearon ER et al (1991) Scrambled exons. Cell 64:607–613

13. Sambrook J, Fritsch EF, Maniatis T (1989) Molecular cloning: a laboratory manual. Spring Harbor Laboratory Press, New York

14. Salzman J (2016) Circular RNA expression: its potential regulation and function. Trends Genet 32:309–316

Chapter 6

Detecting Circular RNAs by RNA Fluorescence In Situ Hybridization

Anne Zirkel and Argyris Papantonis

Abstract

Fluorescence in situ hybridization (FISH) coupled to high-resolution microscopy is a powerful method for analyzing the subcellular localization of RNA. However, the detection of circular RNAs (circRNAs) using microscopy is challenging because the only feature of a circRNA that can be used for the probe design is its junction. Circular RNAs are expressed at varying levels, and for their efficient monitoring by FISH, background fluorescence levels need to be kept low. Here, we describe a FISH protocol coupled to high-precision localizations using a single fluorescently labeled probe spanning the circRNA junction; this allows circRNA detection in mammalian cells with high signal-to-noise ratios.

Key words Single-molecule FISH, Amine chemical labeling, Nascent RNA, Oligonucleotides, Hybridization

1 Introduction

Although discovered decades ago, attention was not drawn to circular RNAs until the last few years (reviewed in ref. [1]). Advances in RNA sequencing technologies and computational analyses enabled the identification of thousands of circRNA species that were also conserved across organisms and taxa [2–6]. Evidence of the functionality and the biological importance of the majority of circRNAs is still under investigation, although some examples were recently described [2, 5, 7], and the field has been rapidly evolving. For any new RNA species discovered, its subcellular localization is always of primary interest. Fluorescence in situ hybridization (FISH) allows the visualization of different RNA species within cells [8], but targeting an RNA that is found in both a linear and circular form can prove challenging. In this chapter, we delineate a universally applicable method to detect circRNAs via a junction-specific probe. CircRNAs are marked by a head-to-tail ligated junction that is not found in any other RNA molecule known to date (with the rare exception of *trans*-splicing) [9]. Hence, this protocol is robust and highly sensitive, and multiple probes, each labeled by a different fluor, can allow for the simultaneous detection of different targets.

2 Materials

Prepare all solutions using RNase-free (DEPC-treated) water. Always wear gloves to avoid sample contamination, and diligently follow all waste disposal regulations when disposing waste materials. Store all solutions and stocks as described below; the hybridization and fixation buffers are always prepared fresh.

1. Probes targeting circRNAs: Oligonucleotides (55-mer), internally modified at (roughly) every tenth thymidine to a 5-C6-amino-2′-dT-modification (IBA, Heidelberg); store unlabeled probes long term at −80°C.

2. Alexa Fluor® Oligonucleotide Amine Labeling Kit (Invitrogen).

3. G-50 columns (GE Healthcare).

4. Microcon-30 column (Millipore).

5. Glass coverslips, strength No. 1 (0.13–0.16 mm; Carl Roth).

6. Glass slides 76 × 26 mm (Carl Roth).

7. Phosphate-buffered saline (PBS): 100 mM Na_2HPO_4, 20 mM KH_2PO_4, 137 mM NaCl, 27 mM KCl, pH 7.4; store at room temperature.

8. Fixation buffer: 1 mL of fixation solution suffices for one well of a 12-well plate; scale up accordingly for multiple wells. For example, for 10 coverslips mix 6 mL of RNase-free water with 1 mL 9% NaCl, 2.5 mL 16% paraformaldehyde (Electron Microscopy Sciences), and 500 μL glacial acetic acid. Always prepare this solution fresh.

9. Pepsin (Sigma Aldrich): A stock solution (1%) can be prepared in RNase-free water and stored at 4°C for ~1 month.

10. 20× SSC: 3 M NaCl, 300 mM sodium citrate, pH 7.0; store at room temperature.

11. Hybridization buffer: The hybridization buffer constitutes 9/10 of the final hybridization mix. It contains 25% formamide, 2× SSC, 200 ng/μL sheared salmon sperm DNA (10 mg/mL; carrier), 5× Denhardt's (0.1% Ficoll 400, 0.1% polyvinylpyrrolidone, 0.1% bovine serum albumin [BSA]), 50 mM phosphate buffer (20 mM KH_2PO_4, 30 mM $KHPO_4*2H_2O$, pH 7.0), and 1 mM ethylenediaminetetraacetic acid (EDTA). Newly opened formamide should be aliquoted and frozen at −80 °C. Always prepare this solution fresh.

12. Rubber cement (Fixogum, Marabu); store at room temperature.

3   Methods

3.1   Probe Design

1. Fluorescently labeled 55-mers are designed to be complementary to the "head-to-tail" circRNA junction [5]; ideally, there should be 22–24 nucleotides complementary to either sides of the junction so as to avoid spurious off-target hybridization. Either control probes can be chosen from published studies, e.g., CDR1-as in neuronal cells [2] (*see* **Note 1**), or intronic probes that detect nascent transcripts from the parental gene locus. For intronic probes it is recommended designing multiple (typically three or four) probes in the same intron to enhance proper detection. The GC content of the probe needs to fall between 40% and 60% (*see* **Note 2**), approximately every tenth nucleotide needs to be a thymidine, and each such thymidine needs to be an amino-modified C6-dT in the final oligo used for labeling [10].

3.2   Labeling of Probes and Purification

1. The modified nucleotides are labeled using the Alexa Fluor® Oligonucleotide Amine Labeling Kit (*see* **Note 3**). First, 15 μg of each oligonucleotide is phenol extracted, ethanol precipitated, and resuspended in 1 μL of RNase-free water. The labeling reaction is performed as per the manufacturer's instructions, except that reaction volumes are reduced in half.

2. Each probe is purified via G-50 columns, ethanol precipitated twice, and washed in 70% ethanol. Each time the absorbance of the 70% ethanol supernatant is checked at the appropriate wavelength (e.g., at 488 nm when labeling with Alexa® 488) to ensure that residual fluors are removed.

3. Reactions are concentrated on a Microcon-30 column as per the manufacturer's instructions, and labeling efficiency is determined from the absorption of each oligo using the extinction coefficients of each fluor and an online calculator (http://www.genelink.com/tools/gl-bdratio.asp). Typically, calculations of 3.5–4.5 fluors per probe are adequate for efficient RNA detection here. Note also that we store labeled probes at a 1 μg/μL concentration at −20 °C for up to 1 year, and unlabeled ones at −80 °C for long term.

3.3   Coverslip Preparation

1. Probe detection in RNA FISH can be significantly enhanced by etching the glass coverslips. Coverslips are treated with 0.1% hydrofluoric acid for 10 min in a sonication bath. Next, rinse coverslips extensively with distilled water (*see* **Note 4**), and store them in 70% until further use.

2. On the day of use, place the coverslips in the tissue culture dishes and wash twice in PBS prior to cell seeding (to facilitate handling of coverslips in tissue culture well, it is advisable to add a drop of medium in each well before placing the coverslip

inside). If your cell type of choice can grow on coverslips directly, avoid coating (e.g., with Matrigel) of coverslips as this can increase unspecific binding of probes and therefore result in higher background fluorescence.

3.4   Cell Fixation

1. The fixative solution should be prepared fresh before each use. Remove cell medium and rinse cells once with PBS.

2. Add enough fixative to fully cover cells, and incubate for 17 min at room temperature.

3. Wash the coverslips once in PBS for 5 min.

4. Add ice-cold 70% ethanol and store the coverslips at least overnight at −20 °C (*see* **Note 5**).

3.5   Permeabilization (with/without Pepsin Digestion)

1. Fixed cells are removed from −20 °C and allowed to recover in PBS for at least 5 min at RT. Depending on the expected localization of the circRNA of interest one needs to decide on the method of choice for the permeabilization (*see* **Note 6**).

    (a) Preserving the cytoplasmic compartment: For preservation of the cytoplasm, a permeabilization step with 0.5% Triton X-100/0.5% saponin for 5–10 min is recommended (*see* **Note 7**). Then, wash coverslips once in PBS before proceeding with post-fixation.

    (b) Focusing on the nuclear compartment only: For circRNAs predicted to be mostly or solely nuclear, a pepsin digestion step can be applied to remove most of the cell's cytoplasm. To this end, a 1% pepsin stock solution is prepared in RNase-free water. The working dilution is 0.01% pepsin that needs to be activated by 10 mM HCl at 37 °C for 3–5 min before the pepsin solution is added to the cells. It is critical to monitor how the digestion progresses under a microscope. Typically, full digestion will not take more than 5 min at room temperature. Pepsin digestion is stopped by washing the solution out with RNase-free water three times (*see* **Note 8**). If pepsin is used, no additional permeabilization is required.

3.6   Post-fixation and Preparation for Hybridization

1. For post-fixation, 3.7% formaldehyde in PBS is added to the cells for 5 min at room temperature, followed by one 10-min wash in PBS.

2. Next, cells are dehydrated prior to hybridization by the addition of 70, 90, and 100% ethanol (3 min each), and then coverslips are air-dried.

3.7   Hybridization

1. Prepare hybridization mix fresh; calculate a total of 20 μL per sample [18 μL hybridization mix + 2 μL probe (25 ng/μL)]. If multiple probes are mixed, decrease the amount of the individual probes accordingly, without adding less than 15 ng in total.

2. Denature the mix at 90 °C for 10 min, and then place immediately on ice. Place 15 μL of the hybridization mix in the middle of a clean glass slide, and inverse a dried coverslip onto the drop using forceps (*see* **Note 9**).

3. The coverslip is sealed using rubber cement, placed in a humid chamber sealed with parafilm (*see* **Note 10**), and incubated at 37 °C overnight. Samples must be protected from direct light.

3.8 Post-hybridization Washing

1. Next day, the rubber cement seal is carefully removed, and coverslips are placed back into a tissue culture dish to be washed three times for 10 min at 37 °C with 2× SSC.

2. Wash once with RNase-free water before DAPI staining for 5 min at RT. Finally, coverslips are dried by touching the edge on a clean tissue, and mounted onto clean glass slides using ProLong® Gold Antifade (Invitrogen).

3. Allow slides to dry overnight protected from light.

3.9 Imaging and High-Precision Localizations

1. Images are recorded on a wide-field fluorescence microscope via a 63× oil objective (Fig. 1; using a Leica system); depending on the expression levels and localization of the target circRNA, not all cells will carry FISH signal (*see* **Note 11**). Critically, to control for signal specificity, RNase R

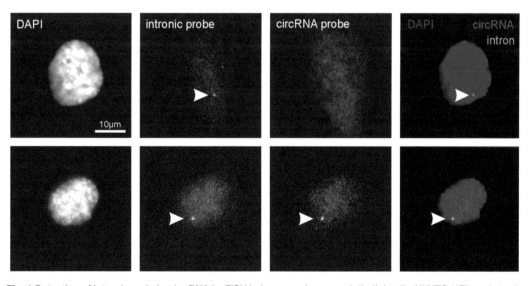

Fig. 1 Detection of intronic and circular RNA by FISH in human primary endothelial cells (HUVECs). Three intronic probes for the parental gene of the circRNA were designed; the targeted intron lies 43 kbp upstream of the exons giving rise to the circRNA. Two typical cells are shown. Upper row: This cell only shows nuclear FISH signal for the intronic probes, indicating the active site of transcription of the parental gene. Lower row: In this cell, specific signals for the circRNA and the intronic probes are detected in the nucleus, in close proximity, indicative of the expression of the nascent transcript and the circRNA, presumably in a co-transcriptional manner

(circRNAs are not degraded; *see* ref. [11] or RNase A (all RNA species are degraded) can be added to cells grown on a coverslip prior to hybridization. The FISH signal emanating from these types of probes yields sub-diffraction spots (*see* Fig. 1); this allows for their high-precision localization using a simple MATLAB plug-in as previously described [12].

4   Notes

1. The probes designed for the CDR1-as are a special case because they do not span the junction. CDR1-as circular RNA can only be detected because it is the major RNA species produced in neuronal tissues or cells from this gene locus.

2. GC content of the probe: Due to the limited options for probe design, one can test different formamide concentrations, if the GC content is outside the recommended range of 40–60%.

3. Multiplexing of multiple probes is feasible. The amine labeling kit is available with different fluorophores. Alternatively, directly labeled probes can be purchased from IBA.

4. Extensive washing of the glass coverslips is needed to remove all residual hydrofluoric acid.

5. Cells can be stored for several days to weeks.

6. If the localization is unknown the permeabilization step (A) and therefore the preservation of the cytoplasm should be tried first. The digestion of the cells with pepsin (B) improves signal-to-noise ratio for nuclear RNAs.

7. Depending on the cell type and the background of the fluorescent probes permeabilization time needs to be tested; for example, for HUVECs 6 min works best.

8. Due to the pepsin treatment many cells and cell parts will become detached. It's critical to stop the reaction when nuclei are still intact but the cytoplasm is mainly removed. Water needs to be added very carefully to stop the reaction. Cell attachment is very fragile at this point.

9. Avoid formation of air bubbles in the hybridization mix when placing the coverslip.

10. For the humid chamber, a paper towel soaked in 2xSSC is placed in the plastic container.

11. circRNA FISH detection needs to be evaluated each time for the signal-to-noise ratio that the particular probe yields in the cell type of interest.

Acknowledgments

This work was supported by a CMMC core funding awarded to A.P., and by a Köln Fortune fellowship awarded to A.Z.

References

1. Cortes-Lopez M, Miura P (2016) Emerging functions of circular RNAs. Yale J Biol Med 89:527–537

2. Memczak S, Jens M, Elefsinioti A, Torti F, Krueger J et al (2013) Circular RNAs are a large class of animal RNAs with regulatory potency. Nature 495:333–338

3. Salzman J, Gawad C, Wang PL, Lacayo N, Brown PO (2012) Circular RNAs are the predominant transcript isoform from hundreds of human genes in diverse cell types. PLoS One 7:e30733

4. Guo JU, Agarwal V, Guo H, Bartel DP (2014) Expanded identification and characterization of mammalian circular RNAs. Genome Biol 15:409

5. Jeck WR, Sharpless NE (2014) Detecting and characterizing circular RNAs. Nat Biotechnol 32:453–461

6. Szabo L, Salzman J (2016) Detecting circular RNAs: bioinformatic and experimental challenges. Nat Rev Genet 17:679–692

7. Yang W, Du WW, Li X, Yee AJ, Yang BB (2016) Foxo3 activity promoted by non-coding effects of circular RNA and Foxo3 pseudogene in the inhibition of tumor growth and angiogenesis. Oncogene 35:3919–3931

8. Itzkovitz S, van Oudenaarden A (2011) Validating transcripts with probes and imaging technology. Nat Methods 8:S12–S19

9. Gingeras TR (2009) Implications of chimaeric non-co-linear transcripts. Nature 461:206–211

10. Wada Y, Ohta Y, Xu M, Tsutsumi S, Minami T et al (2009) A wave of nascent transcription on activated human genes. Proc Natl Acad Sci U S A 106:18357–18361

11. Tan WL, Lim BT, Anene-Nzelu CG, Ackers-Johnson M, Dashi A et al (2017) A landscape of circular RNA expression in the human heart. Cardiovasc Res 113:298–309

12. Larkin JD, Papantonis A, Cook PR, Marenduzzo D (2013) Space exploration by the promoter of a long human gene during one transcription cycle. Nucleic Acids Res 41:2216–2227

Chapter 7

Single-Molecule Fluorescence In Situ Hybridization (FISH) of Circular RNA CDR1as

Christine Kocks, Anastasiya Boltengagen, Monika Piwecka, Agnieszka Rybak-Wolf, and Nikolaus Rajewsky

Abstract

Individual mRNA molecules can be imaged in fixed cells by hybridization with multiple, singly labeled oligonucleotide probes, followed by computational identification of fluorescent signals. This approach, called single-molecule RNA fluorescence in situ hybridization (smRNA FISH), allows subcellular localization and absolute quantification of RNA molecules in individual cells. Here, we describe a simple smRNA FISH protocol for two-color imaging of a circular RNA, CDR1as, simultaneously with an unrelated messenger RNA. The protocol can be adapted to circRNAs that coexist with overlapping, noncircular mRNA isoforms produced from the same genetic locus.

Key words circRNA visualization, circRNA quantification, FISH, Single-molecule detection, In situ hybridization, Absolute quantification of gene expression

1 Introduction

Methods to detect RNA molecules by in situ hybridization are based on protocols that were originally developed in the late 1960s for detection of cellular DNA. They exploit the high stability of RNA–DNA hybrid molecules that form in the presence of formamide, an ionic agent that lowers the melting temperature of DNA double strands [1, 2]. In contrast to DNA, however, target RNA molecules are single stranded, and do not require the harsh melting temperatures and high formamide concentrations needed to open up double-stranded DNA molecules. In the protocol described here, the use of multiple, short DNA oligonucleotide probes with about 45% GC content enables hybridization of target RNA molecules under mild conditions: 37 °C and 10% formamide.

This protocol is based on pioneering work of Robert Singer and colleagues [3–5]. It was further developed to its current form by Raj and Tyagi [6, 7] and was licensed commercially as Stellaris®

Christoph Dieterich and Argyris Papantonis (eds.), *Circular RNAs: Methods and Protocols*, Methods in Molecular Biology, vol. 1724, https://doi.org/10.1007/978-1-4939-7562-4_7, © Springer Science+Business Media, LLC 2018

RNA FISH. It relies on the simple concept of exposing fixed cells or tissues to short DNA oligonucleotides in sufficiently high concentrations to allow pairing with complementary RNA molecules to form stable DNA–RNA hybrids. The probes consist of a pooled set of ~32 to 48 DNA oligos of different sequence, each 20 nucleotides long and labeled with a single fluorophore at its 3′ end (Fig. 1).

The protocol is able to detect single RNA molecules with high specificity (few false positives) and high sensitivity (few false negatives) and does not require signal amplification steps, which tend to render single-molecule detection approaches less quantitative [11, 12]. Two-color FISH targeting different regions in the same transcript molecules (coding region and 3′UTR) yielded a sensitivity of 60–80% (measured as co-localized spots) [6, 8, 13], and the absolute number of RNA spots is generally in good agreement with measurements from quantitative real-time PCR experiments [7, 8, 14].

In mammalian cells, mRNA molecules are about 3000-fold less abundant than protein molecules: NIH 3T3 mouse fibroblasts, for example, express a median of 17 mRNA molecules compared to a median of around 50,000 protein molecules [15]. This ratio explains why, given the physical properties of fluorescent dyes,

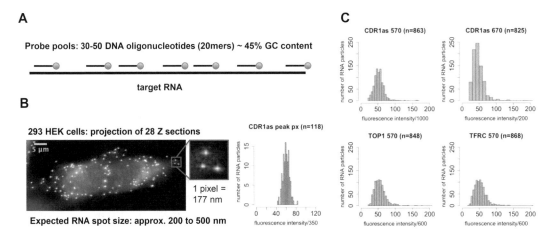

Fig. 1 Single-molecule detection of circRNA CDR1as by RNA FISH. (**a**) The method uses a pooled set of single-stranded DNA oligos of different sequences, each 20 nucleotides long and labeled with a single fluorophore at its 3′ end. A custom oligonucleotide probe set was designed using a freely available algorithm (Stellaris Probe Designer, LGC Biosearch Technologies) [6, 7]. (**b**) RNA FISH of circRNA CDR1as (left) displayed unimodal distribution of peak pixel intensities (right), consistent with single-molecule detection [8]. Peak pixel intensities were determined with open-source software Fiji [9]. (**c**) Magnitude and unimodal distribution of integrated (sum) pixel intensities for circRNA CDR1as are comparable with mRNA detection in the same cells (TOP1, topoisomerase; TFRC, transferrin receptor). Probe sets contained 48 oligonucleotides (CDR1as) or 30 oligonucleotides (TOP1, TFRC). Pixel intensities were measured using the freely available algorithm Localize [10]. Quasar fluorophore type is indicated (570 = Cy3 equivalent; 670 = Cy5 equivalent). (**b, c**), *n* = number of individual cells analyzed

fluorescent signals for mRNA detection with the Stellaris method are much weaker than for protein detection by conventional immunofluorescence. Their relatively low abundance makes it possible to image single RNA molecules as individual, diffraction-limited spots [16]. Thirty to fifty fluorescently labeled oligonucleotides converge onto the same complementary RNA target molecule, and thereby generate a fluorescent, spotlike signal – within the limits of light microscopic resolution (~250 nm) [6, 7] (Fig. 1) – that occurs specifically in the cells of interest and not in controls (Fig. 2). Photobleaching, which is primarily caused by molecular oxygen during the long exposure times required for image acquisition, is reduced by enzymatic oxygen removal [6, 7, 20, 21].

Diffraction-limited spots are identified computationally [6, 7, 10] by a series of steps that involve (1) image acquisition with ~0.25 to 0.3 μm steps in z direction (thus cutting through a spot 2–3 times on average); (2) merging individual z images to maximum-intensity projections; (3) filtering the raw data by a 3D spatial filter (Laplacian of Gaussian), designed to enhance spots of correct size and shape (rapid intensity changes) while removing the background (slowly varying intensity changes); and finally (4) removing particulate noise by counting only signals above a fluorescence intensity threshold (after plotting the number of RNA spots as a function of the threshold value) (Fig. 3a–c). Good image

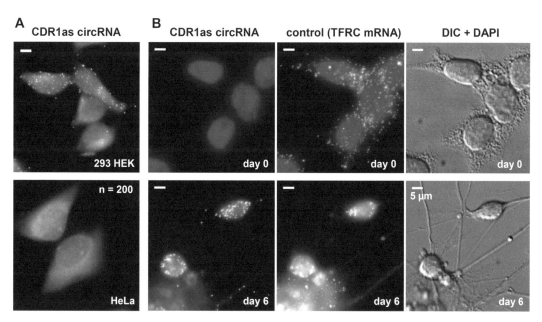

Fig. 2 Examples of specificity controls for CDR1as circRNA detection. (**a**) CircRNA CDR1as is expressed in HEK 293 cells, which are of neural lineage origin [17, 18], but not in epithelial HeLa cells. (**b**) Upper panels: circRNA CDR1as could not be detected in undifferentiated P19 v carcinoma cells (day 0). Lower panels: CDR1as expression 6 days after neuronal differentiation [19]. TFRC mRNA can be detected in both types of cells

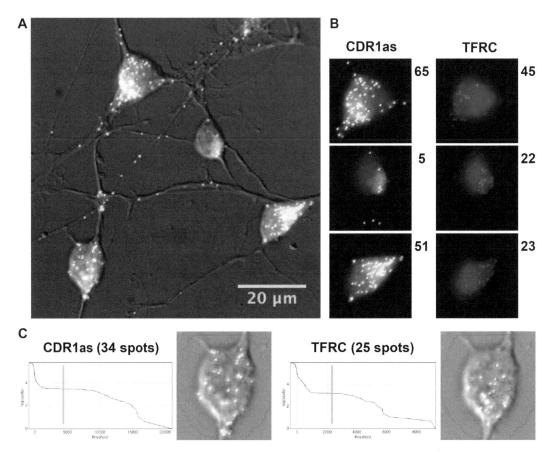

Fig. 3 Localization and quantification of CDR1as circRNA molecules in neurons. (**a**) CircRNA CDR1as (yellow) is localized in cell bodies (soma) and cell extensions (neurites) of P19 neurons in vitro. Transferrin receptor mRNA (TFRC, pink spots) is localized in the nuclear periphery. (**b**) CDR1as expression varies between individual neurons. (**c**) Example of simultaneous RNA spot quantification in two spectrally different fluorescence channels for one individual cell using the freely available software app StarSearch by Marshall Levesque and Arjun Raj, University of Pennsylvania (rajlab.seas.upenn.edu/StarSearch/launch.html). Note that the fluorescence intensity thresholds display plateau-like regions, in which the number of spots detected is relatively insensitive to the threshold value [6, 7]

quality, sufficient for reliable quantification, is indicated by a plateau-like region, in which the spot count is relatively insensitive to the threshold chosen [6, 7] (Fig. 3c).

How do we know that this procedure can detect single RNA molecules? If we assume that the spatial extent of a characteristic globular protein is ~3 to 6 nm in diameter (Bio Number ID101827) and the spatial extent of a characteristic RNA molecule ~40 nm (Bio Number IDs 101827 and 107712) [22–24], it follows that we cannot be sure that a diffraction-limited RNA spot signal of ~250 nm corresponds to a single molecule. In favor of a single-molecule nature of mRNA fluorescent signal detection with the

Stellaris method the following arguments apply [8]: (i) On a molecule-per-cell basis, comparisons with absolute quantification by quantitative real-time PCR were close within the same order of magnitude [8, 14]. (ii) Singer and colleagues [5] calibrated the fluorescence intensities of single-oligonucleotide probes in solution and showed that in yeast cells single-actin mRNA molecules showed expected fluorescence intensities depending on how many probes were bound. (iii) The Tyagi lab used two sets of identical DNA oligos labeled with two spectrally different dyes; they observed no co-localization after injection of a mixture of pre-formed DNA::RNA hybrid molecules into cells [14]. (iv) Furthermore, signal intensities of single mRNA spots were unimodal [14], similar to the results shown in Fig. 1b, c. (v) More corroborating evidence came from super-resolution imaging used to read out sequential combinatorial color barcodes lined up on the same RNA molecule within a single-RNA spot [13].

One should keep in mind, however, that different RNA molecules may behave differently: For example, RNA dimers have been described for Drosophila mRNAs bicoid and oskar, and for retroviral RNAs [25]. Recent evidence indicates that the composition of RNA transport granules in neurons can change over time and in space [8, 26–29] and that mRNA molecules may be inaccessible to smRNA FISH probes due to dense packaging in RNA granules [27]. Removal of proteins by pretreatment with a protease can unmask such RNA molecules.

How do we know that an RNA spot signal is specific? The Stellaris method has an intrinsically high signal-to-noise ratio: signal is generated by convergence of 30–50 fluorophores bound to different oligonucleotides [6, 7]. Stellaris probes consist of complex mixtures of dozens of individual oligonucleotide probes, each of which individually binds to off-targets. However, since binding of individual oligonucleotides contributes only a small fraction of the overall signal, in an ideal scenario, nonspecific binding would only generate a small part of the overall signal and would be unlikely to cause problems. Imaging of mRNA molecules is therefore relatively straightforward, since most mRNAs localize to the cytoplasm and a general idea about their expression levels can be derived from mRNAseq data or from quantitative real-time PCR assays.

By contrast, detection of noncoding RNA molecules poses more of a challenge, because assumptions in terms of expected localization patterns cannot be made, and individual oligonucleotides may generate strong, misleading signals when binding to an abundant or a conspicuously located off-target [30, 31]. In addition, control probe sets against an unrelated or a non-expressed RNA target may give you a good indication of nonspecific signals in general, but will not be informative in terms of specificity of the actual probe set of interest. It is therefore important to perform rigorous controls that are conclusive with respect to the specific probe set of interest. Examples are as follows: (1) cells not expressing the RNA target (such as an unrelated cell line or cell type) (Fig. 2a); (2) transcriptional induction of the target RNA of interest (by induction of differentiation, artificially inducible constructs or drugs) (Fig. 2b); (3) RNAi knockdown of the target RNA [32]; and (4) ideally, use of cells in which the genomic locus or the promoter of the target RNA was deleted. Another, somewhat less practical and more costly possibility is to synthesize two-color probe sets where each second oligo nucleotide is labeled with the other fluorophore (even/odd approach: even-numbered oligos in one color, odd-numbered oligos in another color) [30, 31]. Recent advances in probe labeling may make this approach more affordable [33].

Single-stranded, circular (i.e., covalently closed) RNA molecules are widespread [34, 35], and particularly abundant in mammalian cells [32, 36, 37]. These RNA isoforms are generated by a "back-splicing" reaction, in which the 3′ end of an exon is joined to an upstream 5′ end of an exon, while introns are mostly removed [38–40]. Since they do not have 5′ and 3′ ends, circRNAs escape the regular cellular mRNA turnover mechanisms and are relatively stable compared to the majority of mRNAs or other noncoding RNAs [32]. CircRNAs may carry out distinct biological functions that are different from other RNA molecules. Many circRNAs show tissue- or developmental stage-specific expression [32, 36, 41], making them interesting new targets for molecular imaging.

For the majority of circRNAs, smRNA FISH imaging will be complicated by the simultaneous occurrence of "linear" isoforms with open 5′ and 3′ ends, such as mRNAs, which are generated from the same genomic locus and may coexist in the same cell. Moreover, some genes produce more than one circular isoform, and the ratio of covalently closed (circular) to open ("linear") isoforms and mRNAs can vary in a tissue- or in a context-dependent manner [41]. The well-characterized circRNA CDR1as is exceptional in this respect, since it represents a single dominant isoform: noncircular isoforms from this locus cannot be detected, presumably because CDR1as is very efficiently circularized, or noncircular isoforms are highly unstable [32, 42, 43].

Here we provide a simple protocol to image and quantify CDR1as, a mammalian-specific, noncoding, circular RNA that harbors more than 70 conserved seed matches to the ancient microRNA-7 (miR-7) [32, 43]. CDR1as binds to miR-7 in live cells and can function as a "miRNA sponge" in vivo. Both CDR1as and miR-7 are highly expressed in brain tissues [32, 41, 43]. We detected CDR1as predominantly in the cytoplasm (Fig. 1b) with unimodal spot intensity distributions, suggesting that smRNA FISH signals of CDR1as correspond to single, individual RNA molecules (Fig. 1b, c). The signal is specific, since epithelial cells do not express the molecule (Fig. 2a), and it is specifically induced after neuronal differentiation (Fig. 2b). In neuronal cells, CDR1as occurs in neuronal cell bodies as well as in neuronal cell extensions (Fig. 3a). By two-color fluorescence, we simultaneously imaged transferrin receptor mRNA, which showed a distinct, nonoverlapping localization pattern (Fig. 3b, c). In contrast to transferrin receptor mRNA, CDR1as expression was variable between individual neuronal cells, with RNA particle counts ranging from 5 to 65 or more per cell (Fig. 3b, and data not shown).

To make this protocol more generally applicable to circRNAs that overlap with "linear" mRNAs, it is possible to use the same two-color fluorescence approach presented here by targeting two different probe sets to different regions in the transcript [6] with a signal overlap indicating a circularized and a one-color signal a nonoverlapping region in a "linear" isoform. Variations of this approach have been used to image nascent transcripts at transcription sites and to determine nuclear retention rates of transcripts [44, 45] and to study splicing [46] or to identify splice isoforms [8, 47]. Circularized and noncircularized exons can in this way be distinguished, and their ratios quantified. It should be stressed, however, that any imaging approach for a circRNAs must be backed up by careful molecular analysis of circular and noncircular isoforms, for example by using quantitative real-time PCR assays, or Northern blots combined with RNaseR-mediated degradation of non-covalently closed RNA species, or oligonucleotide-directed RNaseH-mediated cleavage of RNA::DNA duplexes [40, 41, 48].

2 Materials

(See Note 1).

2.1 Equipment

1. Clean 37 °C incubator or dedicated oven for nucleic acid hybridization (see Note 2).

2. A standard high-end wide-field fluorescence microscope equipped with a strong mercury lamp or solid-state white light excitation (Lumencor Sola SE II Light Engine or equivalent), a cooled CCD camera, high-numerical-aperture (Na > 1.3) 60× or 100× oil objectives, an automated stage in Z direction, and image acquisition software (see Note 3). Access to a local server for data backup is desirable.

3. Appropriate filter sets: For two-color FISH with Stellaris probes labeled with Quasar 570 (Cy3 replacement) and Quasar 670 (Cy5 replacement), we use the following filter sets (AHF Analysentechnik AG; wavelength in nm): DAPI HC min bleaching (#F36-513) Ex 387/11 DM 409 Em 447/60; TRITC HC (#F36-503) Ex 543/22 DM 562 Em

593/40; EGFP HC (#F36-525) Ex 472/30 DM 495 Em 520/35; Cy5 HC (#F36-523) Ex 628/40 DM 660 Em 692/40 (*see* **Note 4**).

2.2 Reagents

Reagents should be of purest grade (p. a., or molecular biology grade). All reagents and buffers should be made with nuclease-free, ultrapure water, or bought nuclease free from a trusted supplier. Formaldehyde, formamide, and HCl have to be stored, handled, and disposed of in compliance with safety regulations.

2.3 Acid-Washed Coverslips and Coating Reagents

1. 12-Well plates.

2. 18 mm Ø circle coverslip No. 1 borosilicate glass (for example Thermo Fisher Scientific 10249911 or Roth P233.1): Wash two packages f coverslips (200 pieces) in deionized water, decant. Incubate in 1 M HCl in a glass beaker for 6 h. Agitate gently from time to time. Decant HCl and wash extensively with deionized water. Wash once in ultrapure water, decant. Wash and disinfect in 70% ethanol, decant. Store in 100% ethanol in a small, clean, tightly closed glass flask (wide mouth). Remove with fine forceps and let air-dry before coating and plating cells (*see* **Note 5**).

3. 0.1 mg/mL Poly-D-lysine: Dissolve 5 mg poly-D-lysine (Sigma P6407-5MG) in 50 mL sterile PBS. Store 10 and 1 mL aliquots at −20°C; use diluted at 1:3.3 in PBS (33 μg/mL).

4. 20 μg/mL Laminin: Dilute laminin stock solution (Sigma L2020-1MG; 1–2 mg/mL in Tris-buffered NaCl) to 20 μg/mL in PBS. Store 10 and 1 mL aliquots at −20 °C; use diluted at 1:20.

2.4 Fixation

1. Formaldehyde solution 16% methanol-free EM grade (Polysciences 18814-10, 20 × 10 mL): For 40 mL of 4% formaldehyde fixative containing 1 mM Ca and 1 mM Mg, dispense 26 mL of RNase-free water in a 50-mL Falcon tube. Add 4 mL of 10× PBS. Add 40 μL each of 1 M $CaCl_2$ and $MgCl_2$. Carefully break the neck of a single-use 16% formaldehyde ampule and transfer the content (10 mL) to the Falcon tube. Mix. The pH should be around 7.4; check with pH paper by placing a drop on the pH paper. Filter the fixative solution through a 0.2 μm filter to remove fine particles. Prepare 5 or 10 mL aliquots. Use immediately or keep on ice until needed. Remaining aliquots can be stored at −20 °C for several months (*see* **Note 6**).

2. 1× Dulbecco's PBS supplemented with Ca and Mg; 1 M $MgCl_2$ solution; 1 M $CaCl_2$ solution.

3. 70% Ethanol.

2.5 Hybridization (Day 1)

1. Humidified chamber that seals tightly (can be home-made from plastic containers with a small glass plate to provide a flat surface).

2. 20× SSC (300 mM sodium chloride, 30 mM sodium citrate pH 7).

3. Deionized formamide: Buy the smallest quantity available (100 mL), since formamide oxidizes to formic acid when exposed to air and can go bad. Aliquot in 5 and 1 mL aliquots in polypropylene tubes, close tightly, and store at −20 °C.

4. Dextran sulfate (Sigma D8906-50G).

5. Hybridization buffer (2× SSC, 10% w/v dextran sulfate, 10% formamide): Place 6.5 mL nuclease-free water in a 15 mL polypropylene tube. Add 1 g dextran sulfate. Place at room temperature on an end-over-end rotator for several hours; make sure that dextran sulfate is completely dissolved. Then add 1 mL formamide and 1 mL of 20× SSC. Fill up to 10 mL with water, if necessary. Store in 0.5 or 1 mL aliquots at −20 °C.

6. Wash buffer (2× SSC, 10% formamide): Mix 40 mL water, 5 mL 20× SSC, and 5 mL deionized formamide. Store 10 mL aliquots at −20 °C.

2.6 Washing, DAPI Staining, and Mounting in Oxygen Removal Medium (Day 2)

1. One aliquot of wash buffer, thawed and stored at 4 °C.

2. 4′,6-Diamino-2-phenylindole (DAPI) dilactate (Sigma D9564-10MG): Prepare a 5 mg/mL stock solution by dissolving 10 mg DAPI in 2 mL of water; store in aliquots at −20°C. From this stock solution, prepare a 1:1000 pre-dilution in water (5 μg/mL); store aliquots at −20 °C. Keep one pre-diluted working aliquot at 4 °C. Use at 5 ng/mL final concentration in wash buffer.

3. Glass slides, for example Menzel Superfrost (Thermo Scientific 10143560W90; 76 × 26 mm ISO8037/I white with ground edges, ready to use).

4. 10% Glucose; sterile filtered; 2.5 g for 25 mL; frozen aliquots 1 mL; Roth X997.2.

5. 1 M Tris–HCl pH 8; Ambion AM9855G 500 mL nuclease free.

6. 50 mM Sodium acetate pH ~5: Prepare 600 μL freshly every few weeks: Dilute 3 M sodium acetate solution to 50 mM with ultrapure water (1:60).

7. Glucose oxidase from Aspergillus niger (Sigma G0543-10KU): Store undiluted in aliquots at −20 °C or at 4 °C. Prepare a working stock solution at 3.7 mg/mL in 50 mM sodium acetate pH ~5, and keep at 4 °C. Replace working stock every few weeks.

8. Catalase from bovine liver approx. 10 mg/mL (Sigma C3155-50MG): Store aliquots at 4 °C (cannot be frozen). Contains crystals, therefore mix mildly before use, in order to disperse crystals uniformly. Replace aliquots periodically, as they tend to get contaminated easily.

9. Clear transparent finger nail polish: Fast-drying nail polish base works well. Make sure to avoid "volume-enhancing" nail polish.

3   Methods

3.1   Design and Preparation of Probes

1. Design your probe sets using the free Stellaris probe designer (LGC Biosearch Technologies web site; developed by Arjun Raj), which optimizes the GC content of the individual DNA oligonucleotides to around 45%. Create a login name and password and follow the stepwise instructions. We use default settings (20mer probes with a minimum of 2 nt spacing) and the highest species-specific masking level that allows placing a minimum of 32 probes that specifically target the RNA transcript under investigation. Replace unwanted target regions by "n" for specific nucleotides (for example areas around splice sites or repeat regions). Copy the output list of probes from the Stellaris probe designer to an Excel sheet and run a BLAT search. Eliminate individual oligonucleotide probes that match other genomic locations, or bind to overlapping regions in your target locus. It is useful to keep an electronic documentation of these procedures and their results (*see* **Note 7**).

2. Order probe sets (5 nmol) with appropriate fluorophores that match the fluorescence filters in your microscope. For two-color RNA FISH experiments, we use Quasar 570 (Cy3 replacement) and 670 (Cy5 replacement), DAPI as nuclear counterstain, the EGFP channel to control for autofluorescent spots, and the DIC or bright-field channel for cell outlines and as reference focus plane (*see* **Note 8**).

3. Probe sets arrive as a pool of DNA oligonucleotides in dry, lyophilized form (5 nmol; sufficient for up to 400 experiments). For a probe stock of 12.5 μM concentration, dissolve in 400 μL Tris 10 mM EDTA 1 mM pH 8 buffer. Shield and protect probes from bright day- or sunlight. Mix well by pipetting, let stand on ice for 5 min, and mix again by vortexing. Centrifuge at maximum speed in a tabletop centrifuge at 4 °C for 5 min, transfer supernatant to a new microcentrifuge tube (take care not to disturb the pellet), and aliquot: 7×50 μL (for long-term storage) and 50×1 μL (single-use aliquots). Use unique probe identifiers and label tube tops. Probes stored at −80 °C are good for several years.

3.2 Seed, Fix, and Permeabilize Adherent Cells (Flp-In T-Rex 293 HEK Cells)

(*See* **Note 9**).

1. Place one dry, acid-washed cover glass per well in a 12-well plate. Coat cover glass with a 6:3:1 mixture of PBS/poly-D-lysine/laminin for 10 min at room temperature. Wash two times with PBS to remove excess coating. (You can store coated cover glasses at 4 °C overnight.)

2. Seed 2×10^5 logarithmically growing cells in 1 mL growth medium per well; grow for at least 24 h. Cells should be semi-confluent for easier imaging and quantification.

3. Thaw an aliquot of fixation solution (4% formaldehyde in PBS with 1 mM Ca and Mg).

4. Place cells on ice, remove supernatant, and wash cells once with PBS containing 1 mM Ca and Mg. Remove supernatant and gently add 1 mL fixative per well. Remove from ice and incubate at room temperature for 10 min.

5. Remove fixative, and wash with 1 mL cold PBS.

6. Transfer cells back to ice. Remove supernatant and add 2 mL per well of ice-cold 70% ethanol.

7. Cells can be stored in 70% ethanol at 4 °C for weeks to months (*see* **Note 10**).

3.3 Hybridize RNAs (Day 1)

1. Thaw an aliquot of hybridization buffer (1 mL) and wash buffer (10 mL). (This can be done conveniently overnight at 4 °C.)

2. Remove an aliquot of probe solution (12.5 μM) from −80 °C. Thaw, mix, and collect at the bottom of the tube by a brief spin. Place on ice.

3. Prepare a 2× probe dilution at 100 nM concentration by adding 125 μL of hybridization buffer to 1 μL of probe stock (*see* **Note 11**).

4. Transfer four cover glasses to 70% ethanol placed in the first row of a fresh 12-well plate on ice.

5. One by one, remove the 70% ethanol storage solution and add 1 mL of wash buffer. Transfer plate to room temperature and let stand for 2–5 min (longer is fine).

6. Assemble an airtight humid chamber; we use a flat transparent plastic box with a small glass plate (for flat surface) onto which a clean piece of parafilm is placed. Mark the positions with a cross in the middle of the parafilm with a felt pen marker, and mark the four quadrants 1–4.

7. Place into the four quadrants 50 μL each, processing one cover glass after another: (1) a 25 μL of 2× probe dilution A, followed by 25 μL of 2× probe dilution B (two-color FISH); (2) 25 μL of 2× probe solution A, followed by 25 μL hybridization solution (single-color FISH control); (3) 25 μL of 2× probe solu-

tion B, followed by 25 µL hybridization solutions (single-color FISH control); and (4) 50 µL hybridization solution (no probe control). Remove cover glass from wash buffer, one by one; remove excess fluid by dipping the edge of the cover glass onto a lint-free Kimwipe; and place – cells facing downwards – onto the 50 µL droplet.

8. Moisten a Kimwipe with tap water and place in the humid chamber taking care that the moist Kimwipe does not touch any of the cover glasses.

9. Close humid chamber tightly to prevent evaporation and place in a 37 °C incubator overnight. Place wash buffer at 4 °C. Hybridization takes at least 4 h, and can be done for up to 16 h. Hybridizing overnight gives you a full day of imaging.

3.4 Washing and DAPI Staining (Day 2)

1. The next day, float the cover glasses off the parafilm by slowly adding 200 µL of wash buffer with a P200 micropipettor, so that the fluid gets sucked under the cover glass by capillary action (*see* **Note 12**).

2. Place 1 mL wash buffer in four wells of the second row of the 12-well plate from day 1. Lift cover glasses off parafilm (this should be very easy at this step), dip edge onto a Kimwipe, and transfer cover glass to 12-well plate (cell side up).

3. Incubate at 37 °C for 30 min. Shorter washes will prevent the oligos from diffusing out of the cells and may give high background. Washing longer (up to several hours) is no problem.

4. Prepare 5 mL of wash buffer containing 5 ng/mL DAPI (dilute DAPI stock solution 1:1000).

5. After 30 min, remove wash buffer and replace with 1 ml of wash buffer containing 5 ng/mL DAPI. Return to 37 °C and wash and stain for 30 min.

6. Prepare 10 mL of 2× SSC solution.

7. Remove wash buffer and replace with 1 ml of 2× SSC. Place samples on ice. Samples can be kept several hours to overnight at 4 °C.

3.5 Mounting in Oxygen Removal Buffer (Day 2)

1. Keep all solutions and buffers on ice.

2. Thaw an aliquot of 10% sterile glucose solution (0.5 mL).

3. Prepare 5 mL of GLOX buffer: To 4.25 mL of ultrapure water, add 500 µL 20× SSC, 200 µL 10% glucose, and 50 µL of 1 M Tris–HCL pH 8. Vortex and transfer 1 mL of GLOX buffer to a new microcentrifuge tube. The remainder of GLOX buffer is used to equilibrate the samples (1 mL per well).

4. Prepare GLOX buffer plus enzymes (oxygen removal medium): To 1 mL of GLOX buffer from **step 3**, add 10 µL of glucose oxidase working stock (3.7 mg/mL in 50 mM sodium acetate

pH ~5) and 10 μL of gently mixed catalase stock solution, and mix gently.

5. Remove 2×SSC from cells, add 1 mL GLOX buffer per sample, and transfer to room temperature. Let equilibrate for 1–2 min (or longer).

6. Use a lint-free Kimwipe to wipe a glass slide with 70% ethanol, mark the frosted part with pencil, and place a 15 μL droplet of GLOX buffer with enzymes in the center of the dry slide.

7. Remove cover glass from equilibration buffer, dip edge on a Kimwipe to remove excess liquid, and place cell side down onto the oxygen removal medium. Repeat **steps 6–7** for each sample.

8. Gently and carefully blot away excess fluid. Seal edges of coverslip with nail polish, let dry, and then carefully wash the surface of the cover glass with ultrapure water to remove salt and glucose crystals. Blot dry. Take care to not accidentally move the coverslip at this step, as this dislodges cells and molecules.

9. Transfer slides to a plastic tray on ice. Keep samples in the dark until ready for same-day imaging.

3.6   Imaging (Day 2)

1. For reproducible and quantitative results, imaging must be done on the same day (*see* **Note 13**).

2. Focus on cell extensions in the DIC or bright-field channel. Move focus one or two Z steps below (0.3–0.6 μm). Set the lower and upper limits. For HEK cells, acquire 30 Z sections in 0.3 μm steps in the order: Cy5, Cy3, EGPF, DAPI, and DIC. Exposure times vary depending on exact equipment, cells, and probes, but typically require around 1–3 s (Cy5 channel), 0.5–2 s (Cy3 channel), 0.25–0.5 s (EGFP channel), and 50 ms (DAPI channel). Use autoexposure for DIC or bright field, and then fix exposure time manually to keep it constant throughout your experiment (*see* **Note 14**).

3. What to expect: True RNA signals should fulfill the following criteria: Fluorescent signals corresponding to mRNA molecules should be clearly visible above background (signal-to-background ratio of ~2) [49] as discrete, diffraction-limited spots of about 200–500 nm [6, 7], predominantly in the cytoplasm (Fig. 1b). Thus, one RNA spot will show up in 2–3 z sections of 0.3 μm. Specific signals should only appear in the appropriate fluorescence channel, not in the EGFP or any other channel. Signals corresponding to circular RNAs depend on the nature of the circRNA imaged. Similar to the majority of circRNAs [36, 37], circRNA CDR1as is predominantly located in the cytoplasm, and in this respect behaves like an mRNA molecule. Brighter and larger RNA signals in the nucleus typically correspond to transcription start sites: nascent

RNA molecules are still attached to polymerase II molecules and are thought to accumulate at the site of transcription giving rise to larger RNA agglomerates. The detection of transcription start sites depends on transcriptional burst frequency and burst size [44, 50, 51], and because not all cells are transcriptionally active at the same time, transcription start sites will be visible only in a few cells [6, 7].

3.7 Image Processing

1. Export images in monochrome as TIFF files.

2. Process images using the freely available imaging software Fiji (https://fiji.sc) [9]:

    Move images to stacks (Image/Stacks/Images to Stack; Image/Stacks/Tools/Stack Sorter). Merge z images (Image/Stack/Z Project …) using maximum-intensity projections for the Cy5, Cy3, and EGFP channels; choose one z plane image for DAPI (center of nucleus) and one z plane for DIC/bright field (focused on cell extensions). Generate composite two-color overlays (Image/Color/Merge Channels …) for DAPI (blue) and the Cy5 channel (gray), DAPI and the Cy3 channel (gray), and DAPI and the DIC/bright-field channel (gray) (*see* **Note 15**).

3.8 RNA Spot Quantification

1. For RNA spot quantification we use a regular web browser with a freely available JAVA-based software app (StarSearch) developed by Marshall Levesque and Arjun Raj, University of Pennsylvania (*see* [6, 7] for an explanation of the underlying principles) (*see* **Note 16**).

2. Import images into StarSearch. The program will automatically recognize the image type (RNA, nucleus, transmission) through the file names. At the same time in Fiji, keep a color merge between DAPI and your two fluorescent images open. This will allow you to visually inspect your cells in parallel to the quantification process.

3. Click on the first image, maximize the window, and encircle the outlines of a cell. Click: "Process". Compare the spot assignment with your image and modify the threshold, if necessary. Approve the spot count (*see* **Note 17**).

4. Repeat **step 3** for every cell to be quantified. When all cells are processed, make a screenshot of the View controls window to document which cell corresponds to which number in your exported Excel list. Include a typical histogram (spot count versus threshold). Then press "Export data" and rename the Excel results file. Save file to an image quantification folder together with the screenshots.

5. Repeat **steps 3–4** for each image to be analyzed. In Excel, use SUM, AVERAGE, and STDEV functions for each channel.

For robust quantification, proceed until you have quantified about 200 cells. For export into R for further statistical analysis, save file in csv format.

---

4   Notes

1. Before you start with smRNA FISH, visit Arjun Raj's smRNA FISH website: https://sites.google.com/site/singlemoleculernafish/. It is a great resource with abundant background information, protocols, troubleshooting, and answers to many FAQs that cover all aspects of the method.

2. We use a regular molecular biology lab bacterial incubator for molecular cloning and place a clean aluminum tray in it (for even temperature distribution), onto which we place the samples in a tightly sealed, humid chamber.

3. It is important to pay attention to the final spatial resolution of your images, which is primarily a function of the objective (60× or 100×) and the physical pixel size of the CCD sensor in your camera: the resulting resolution should exceed the diffraction limit (thus be less than ~250 nm) [11, 45]. In practice, we were able to obtain good, quantifiable images at a resolution of 177 and 220 nm per pixel with a Keyence BZ-9000 and a Nikon Ti-E inverted microscope, respectively, with Nikon plan apochromat 60× oil objectives (NA 1.4), but this may be setup-specific. RNA spots may be more easily identified computationally, when images are taken with a 100× oil objective [7]. Confocal laser scanning microscopes typically will not work, because the fluorescence signals are too weak and the laser will bleach them before all scans of a cell can be completed. Make sure that you can detect signals with a wide-field fluorescence microscope before using a confocal. By contrast, spinning disk confocal microscopes work well, especially with tissue sections, as they allow imaging in deeper tissue layers [49].

4. Stellaris probe sets are available with a broad choice of labeling fluorophores and other filter combinations will work. Consult your microscope manufacturer for guidance on suitable fluorophores in accordance with your microscope setup and fluorescent light source. Many manufacturers provide trial fluorescence filters without charge. However, be sure to run the "bleedthrough" controls suggested below to exclude the possibility that your signals "cross talk" into another channel under your imaging conditions [6, 7].

5. Do not flame, because cover glasses become brittle and are prone to break later during handling. 12-Well plates with dispensed cover glasses can be prepared ahead of time; store dust free.

6. Alternatively, for convenience, you can use 37% formaldehyde stabilized with 10–15% methanol (formalin; ACS reagent grade) (for example 100 g Fisher Scientific/Acros Organics 10299980). Check the solution for precipitates before use, and either dissolve these by warming the solution or remove by filtering through a 0.45 μm filter. Dilute in PBS to 3.7% and supplement with 1 mM Mg and Ca.

7. A frequent cause of failure is that the target RNA is expressed at too low levels. It is hard to reliably identify RNA molecules that are expressed at less than 5–10 molecules per cell. We recommend starting with well-expressed RNA molecules 20–200 molecules per cell. If no other information on the expression level is available, an indication is RPKM/FPKM (reads/fragments per kilobase per million) counts from next-generation mRNA sequencing data: As a very crude rule of thumb, one RPKM/FPKM corresponds very roughly to about 0.5–5 mRNA molecules per cell depending on the cell type and size [52, 53]. For shorter target RNAs, a trade-off between number of probes and uniformity of GC content arises, and it may be more productive to optimize GC content of the probes to 45%, over placing more probes on a target [7]. Further tips on probe design can be found here [44, 47, 54].

8. It is important to use a well, yet not too highly, expressed mRNA as a positive control. We found TFRC and TOP1 very useful, because they are housekeeping genes that are expressed in many cell types at around 50–70 molecules per cell. Probe sets directed against GAPDH or actin can be useful for initial setup of Stellaris smRNA FISH, but are too highly expressed for quantification.

9. This part of the protocol works well for HEK cells, but it is cell line-specific and needs to be optimized for different cells. Growth and plating conditions should be rigorously standardized for reproducible results [55]. Establish and write a cell line-specific protocol for your cells of interest.

10. In order to prevent ethanol evaporation, seal plates carefully and tightly with parafilm. Note: Cells may not fall dry at any point during the fixation procedure: Process up to four cover glasses (not more) in parallel.

11. In general, we had good success with probe concentrations around 50–100 nM final concentration. For each new probe set, prepare several dilutions to determine the optimal working concentration empirically. Addition of (final) 0.4% SDS (from a 10% SDS stock solution) to the hybridization buffer enhances probe signal relative to background, probably either by increasing probe access to target RNAs or by facilitating diffusion of unbound probes out of the cells. In neurons, it

may be necessary to also apply a brief protease pre-hybridization treatment (0.1 mg/mL pepsin (Sigma P7012), 10 mM HCl in water, pH 2.5 for 45–60 s) to fully unmask tightly condensed RNA particles in granules to make them available for hybridization [27, 28].

12. This step takes some practice. However, it helps to prevent cell damage that would occur, if you tried lifting the coverslips without additional fluid (cells would get ripped off due to negative pressure), and serves as a pre-wash step.

13. Cells mounted in this oxygen removal medium are good for only about 2-h imaging at room temperature. The reason may be that the gluconic acid generated during oxygen scavenging acidifies the medium [21]. This can be prevented by increasing Tris buffer concentration to 50 mM [56]. To further enhance the oxygen radical scavenging activity of the imaging medium, TROLOX, an antioxidant vitamin A analog can be included at 2 mM [45, 49, 57, 58]. Keep samples on ice when not imaged. You can move samples back and forth for repeated imaging, but make sure that samples warm to room temperature before taking pictures. Alternatively, one can use Vectashield mounting medium [47, 54], although in our hands this compromises reliable quantification of smRNA FISH signals, as observed previously [7].

14. Acquire images in monochrome mode preferably at 16- or 12-bit image depth. Typically, using no electronic gain works best, as images become too noisy with gain. However, this is dependent on exact camera type and other equipment (objective, light source). It is also important to acquire images in a sequential order in which the most critical imaging channels are used first (smFISH acquisition: weaker or more sensitive fluorophore first), then autofluorescence monitoring (FITC channel), then DAPI, and bright field last [45, 49]. For rendering cell outlines, it is possible to combine smRNA FISH with F-actin staining using Alexa Fluor 488-phalloidin or to use a FITC-anti-E-cadherin antibody [49].

15. Macros can be generated with the help of the "command recorder" function in order to automate the repetitive steps. As an alternative to Fiji, Image J (https://imagej.nih.gov/ij) [59] as well as other imaging software can be used. However, we noticed with commercial software that maximum-intensity projections can differ and compromise quantification by StarSearch (*see* below). Grayscale works best for visualizing RNA spots, especially when signals are weak. Spotlike signals can be artificially "dilated" by two pixels for better visualization in qualitative images [29].

16. There are other free image analysis software options: The algorithm Localize [10] provides spatial coordinates for each RNA molecule spot, in addition to sum pixel intensities and spot counts and is implemented on a freely available IDL virtual machine (ITT Visual Information Systems). FISH Quant (https://bitbucket.org/muellerflorian/fish_quant) [60] and ImageM [49] are suitable for automated image analysis, but require a MATHLAB-graphical interface and license.

17. For robust RNA spot quantification, the quality of your images is critical. You should be able to see a plateau, in which the actual spot count stays relatively stable [6, 7]. For good images, of sufficient quality to be quantified, a plateau is readily apparent, and oftentimes the automatic threshold settings suggested by the StarSearch app can be taken without further modification.

Acknowledgments

This work was supported by the Deutsche Forschungsgemeinschaft [RA838/5-1 to N.R.] and the Berlin Institute of Health [CRG2aTP7 to N. R.]. We thank Arjun Raj and our BIMSB colleagues Alexander Loewer, Dhana Friedrich, Stefan Preibisch, and Marcel Schilling for discussions and advice.

References

1. Gall JG, Pardue ML (1969) Formation and detection of RNA–DNA hybrid molecules in cytological preparations. Proc Natl Acad Sci U S A 63:378–383

2. John HA, Birnstiel ML, Jones KW (1969) RNA-DNA hybrids at the cytological level. Nature 223:582–587

3. Singer RH, Ward DC (1982) Actin gene expression visualized in chicken muscle tissue culture by using in situ hybridization with a biotinated nucleotide analog. Proc Natl Acad Sci U S A 79:7331–7335

4. Lawrence JB, Singer RH (1986) Intracellular localization of messenger RNAs for cytoskeletal proteins. Cell 45:407–415

5. Femino AM (1998) Visualization of single RNA transcripts in situ. Science 280:585–590. https://doi.org/10.1126/science.280.5363.585

6. Raj A, van den Bogaard P, Rifkin SA et al (2008) Imaging individual mRNA molecules using multiple singly labeled probes. Nat Methods 5:877–879. https://doi.org/10.1038/nmeth.1253

7. Raj A, Tyagi S (2010) Detection of individual endogenous RNA transcripts in situ using multiple singly labeled probes. Methods Enzymol 472:365–386. https://doi.org/10.1016/S0076-6879(10)72004-8

8. Batish M, van den Bogaard P, Kramer FR, Tyagi S (2012) Neuronal mRNAs travel singly into dendrites. Proc Natl Acad Sci U S A 109:4645–4650. https://doi.org/10.1073/pnas.1111226109

9. Schindelin J, Arganda-Carreras I, Frise E et al (2012) Fiji: an open-source platform for biological-image analysis. Nat Methods 9:676–682. https://doi.org/10.1038/nmeth.2019

10. Trcek T, Chao JA, Larson DR et al (2012) Single-mRNA counting using fluorescent in situ hybridization in budding yeast. Nat Protoc 7:408–419. https://doi.org/10.1038/nprot.2011.451

11. Itzkovitz S, van Oudenaarden A (2011) Validating transcripts with probes and imaging technology. Nat Methods 8:S12–S19. https://doi.org/10.1038/nmeth.1573

12. Gaspar I, Ephrussi A (2015) Strength in numbers: quantitative single-molecule RNA detection assays. WIREs Dev Biol 4:135–150. https://doi.org/10.1002/wdev.170

13. Lubeck E, Cai L (2012) Single-cell systems biology by super-resolution imaging and combinatorial labeling. Nat Methods 9:743–748. https://doi.org/10.1038/nmeth.2069

14. Vargas DY, Raj A, Marras SAE et al (2005) Mechanism of mRNA transport in the nucleus. Proc Natl Acad Sci U S A 102:17008–17013. https://doi.org/10.1073/pnas.0505580102

15. Schwanhäusser B, Busse D, Li N et al (2011) Global quantification of mammalian gene expression control. Nature 473:337–342. https://doi.org/10.1038/nature10098

16. Femino A, Fogarty K, Lifshitz LM et al (2003) Visualization of single molecules of mRNA in situ. Methods Enzymol 361:245–304. https://doi.org/10.1016/S0076-6879(03)61015-3

17. Shaw G, Morse S, Ararat M, Graham FL (2002) Preferential transformation of human neuronal cells by human adenoviruses and the origin of HEK 293 cells. FASEB J 16:869–871. https://doi.org/10.1096/fj.01-0995fje

18. Lin Y-C, Boone M, Meuris L et al (2014) Genome dynamics of the human embryonic kidney 293 lineage in response to cell biology manipulations. Nat Commun 5:4767. https://doi.org/10.1038/ncomms5767

19. Nakayama Y, Wada A, Inoue R et al (2014) A rapid and efficient method for neuronal induction of the P19 embryonic carcinoma cell line. J Neurosci Methods 227:100–106. https://doi.org/10.1016/j.jneumeth.2014.02.011

20. Benesh RE, Benesh R (1953) Enzymatic removal of oxygen for polarography and related methods. Science 118:447–448

21. Ha T, Tinnefeld P (2012) Photophysics of fluorescent probes for single-molecule biophysics and super-resolution imaging. Annu Rev Phys Chem 63:595–617. https://doi.org/10.1146/annurev-physchem-032210-103340

22. Milo R, Jorgensen P, Moran U et al (2010) BioNumbers—the database of key numbers in molecular and cell biology. Nucleic Acids Res 38:D750–D753. https://doi.org/10.1093/nar/gkp889

23. Phillips R, Kondev J, Theriot J, Garcia H (2012) Physical biology of the cell, 2nd edn. Garland Science, London and New York

24. Milo R, Phillips R (2015) Cell biology by the numbers. Garland Science, London and New York

25. Jambor H, Brunel C, Ephrussi A (2011) Dimerization of oskar 3' UTRs promotes hitchhiking for RNA localization in the Drosophila oocyte. RNA 17:2049–2057. https://doi.org/10.1261/rna.2686411

26. Park HY, Lim H, Yoon YJ et al (2014) Visualization of dynamics of single endogenous mRNA labeled in live mouse. Science 343: 422–424. https://doi.org/10.1126/science.1239200

27. Buxbaum AR, Wu B, Singer RH (2014) Single β-actin mRNA detection in neurons reveals a mechanism for regulating its translatability. Science 343:419–422. https://doi.org/10.1126/science.1242939

28. Akbalik G, Schuman EM (2014) Molecular biology. mRNA, live and unmasked. Science 343:375–376. https://doi.org/10.1126/science.1249623

29. Buxbaum AR, Yoon YJ, Singer RH, Park HY (2015) Single-molecule insights into mRNA dynamics in neurons. Trends Cell Biol 25: 468–475. https://doi.org/10.1016/j.tcb.2015.05.005

30. Cabili MN, Dunagin MC, McClanahan PD et al (2015) Localization and abundance analysis of human lncRNAs at single-cell and single-molecule resolution. Genome Biol 16:20. https://doi.org/10.1038/nmeth.2589

31. Dunagin M, Cabili MN, Rinn J, Raj A (2014) Methods Mol Biol 1262:3–19. https://doi.org/10.1007/978-1-4939-2253-6_1

32. Memczak S, Jens M, Elefsinioti A et al (2013) Circular RNAs are a large class of animal RNAs with regulatory potency. Nature 495:333–338. https://doi.org/10.1038/nature11928

33. Gaspar I, Wippich F, Ephrussi A (2017) Enzymatic production of single molecule FISH and RNA capture probes. RNA 23(10): 1582–1591. https://doi.org/10.1261/rna.061184.117

34. Salzman J (2016) Circular RNA expression: its potential regulation and function. Trends Genet 32:309–316. https://doi.org/10.1016/j.tig.2016.03.002

35. Ebbesen KK, Hansen TB, Kjems J (2016) Insights into circular RNA biology. RNA Biol:1–11. https://doi.org/10.1080/15476286.2016.1271524

36. Salzman J, Gawad C, Wang PL et al (2012) Circular RNAs are the predominant transcript isoform from hundreds of human genes in diverse cell types. PLoS One 7:e30733. https://doi.org/10.1371/journal.pone.0030733

37. Jeck WR, Sorrentino JA, Wang K et al (2013) Circular RNAs are abundant, conserved, and associated with ALU repeats. RNA 19: 141–157. https://doi.org/10.1261/rna.035667.112

38. Ashwal-Fluss R, Meyer M, Pamudurti NR et al (2014) circRNA biogenesis competes with pre-mRNA splicing. Mol Cell 56:55–66. https://doi.org/10.1016/j.molcel.2014.08.019

39. Zhang X-O, Wang H-B, Zhang Y et al (2014) Complementary sequence-mediated exon circularization. Cell 159:134–147. https://doi.org/10.1016/j.cell.2014.09.001

40. Starke S, Jost I, Rossbach O et al (2015) Exon circularization requires canonical splice signals. Cell Rep 10:103–111. https://doi.org/10.1016/j.celrep.2014.12.002

41. Rybak-Wolf A, Stottmeister C, Glažar P et al (2015) Circular RNAs in the mammalian brain are highly abundant, conserved, and dynamically expressed. Mol Cell 58:870–885. https://doi.org/10.1016/j.molcel.2015.03.027

42. Hansen TB, Wiklund ED, Bramsen JB et al (2011) miRNA-dependent gene silencing involving Ago2-mediated cleavage of a circular antisense RNA. EMBO J 30:4414–4422. https://doi.org/10.1038/emboj.2011.359

43. Hansen TB, Jensen TI, Clausen BH et al (2013) Natural RNA circles function as efficient microRNA sponges. Nature 495:384–388. https://doi.org/10.1038/nature11993

44. Bahar Halpern K, Caspi I, Lemze D et al (2015) Nuclear retention of mRNA in mammalian tissues. Cell Rep 13:2653–2662. https://doi.org/10.1016/j.celrep.2015.11.036

45. Bahar Halpern K, Itzkovitz S (2016) Single molecule approaches for quantifying transcription and degradation rates in intact mammalian tissues. Methods 98:134–142. https://doi.org/10.1016/j.ymeth.2015.11.015

46. Vargas DY, Shah K, Batish M et al (2011) Single-molecule imaging of transcriptionally coupled and uncoupled splicing. Cell 147:1054–1065. https://doi.org/10.1016/j.cell.2011.10.024

47. Orjalo AV, Johansson HE (2016) Stellaris® RNA fluorescence in situ hybridization for the simultaneous detection of immature and mature long noncoding RNAs in adherent cells. Methods Mol Biol 1402:119–134. https://doi.org/10.1007/978-1-4939-3378-5_10

48. Jeck WR, Sharpless NE (2014) Detecting and characterizing circular RNAs. Nat Biotechnol 32:453–461. https://doi.org/10.1038/nbt.2890

49. Lyubimova A, Itzkovitz S, Junker JP et al (2013) Single-molecule mRNA detection and counting in mammalian tissue. Nat Protoc 8:1743–1758. https://doi.org/10.1038/nprot.2013.109

50. Halpern KB, Tanami S, Landen S et al (2015) Bursty gene expression in the intact mammalian liver. Mol Cell 58:147–156. https://doi.org/10.1016/j.molcel.2015.01.027

51. Ben-Moshe S, Itzkovitz S (2016) Bursting through the cell cycle. Elife 5:e14953. https://doi.org/10.7554/eLife.14953

52. Mortazavi A, Williams BA, McCue K et al (2008) Mapping and quantifying mammalian transcriptomes by RNA-Seq. Nat Methods 5:621–628. https://doi.org/10.1038/nmeth.1226

53. Kellis M, Wold B, Snyder MP et al (2014) Defining functional DNA elements in the human genome. Proc Natl Acad Sci U S A 111:6131–6138. https://doi.org/10.1073/pnas.1318948111

54. Coassin SR, Orjalo AV, Semaan SJ, Johansson HE (2014) Simultaneous detection of nuclear and cytoplasmic RNA variants utilizing Stellaris® RNA fluorescence in situ hybridization in adherent cells. Methods Mol Biol 1211:189–199. https://doi.org/10.1007/978-1-4939-1459-3_15

55. Batish M, Raj A, Tyagi S (2011) Single molecule imaging of RNA in situ. Methods Mol Biol 714:3–13. https://doi.org/10.1007/978-1-61779-005-8_1

56. Shi X, Lim J, Ha T (2010) Acidification of the oxygen scavenging system in single-molecule fluorescence studies: in situ sensing with a ratiometric dual-emission probe. Anal Chem 82:6132–6138. https://doi.org/10.1021/ac1008749

57. Rasnik I, McKinney SA, Ha T (2006) Nonblinking and long-lasting single-molecule fluorescence imaging. Nat Methods 3:891–893. https://doi.org/10.1038/nmeth934

58. Cordes T, Vogelsang J, Tinnefeld P (2009) On the mechanism of Trolox as antiblinking and antibleaching reagent. J Am Chem Soc 131:5018–5019. https://doi.org/10.1021/ja809117z

59. Schneider CA, Rasband WS, Eliceiri KW (2012) NIH Image to ImageJ: 25 years of image analysis. Nat Methods 9:671–675

60. Mueller F, Senecal A, Tantale K et al (2013) FISH-quant: automatic counting of transcripts in 3D FISH images. Nat Methods 10:277–278. https://doi.org/10.1038/nmeth.2406

Chapter 8

A Highly Efficient Strategy for Overexpressing circRNAs

Dawei Liu, Vanessa Conn, Gregory J. Goodall, and Simon J. Conn

Abstract

Circular RNAs (circRNAs) constitute an emerging class of widespread, abundant, and evolutionarily conserved noncoding RNA. They play important and diverse roles in cell development, growth, and tumorigenesis, but functions of the majority of circRNAs remain enigmatic. In order to investigate circRNA function it is necessary to manipulate its expression. While various standard approaches exist for circRNA knockdown, here we present cloning vectors for simplifying the laborious process of cloning circRNAs to achieve high-efficiency overexpression in mammalian cell lines.

Key words Circular RNA, RNA splicing, Expression constructs, RT-PCR

1 Introduction

Circular RNAs (circRNAs) are covalent circles of single-stranded RNA that arise from noncanonical, back splicing of pre-mRNAs and noncoding RNAs [1, 2]. Due to technical limitations of traditional methods for analyzing RNA sequencing data, circular RNAs were largely overlooked until recently. These advances have shown that circRNAs are highly abundant, gene specific, cell type specific, and developmentally regulated in all eukaryotes indicating that they might be involved in many biological processes and are likely to have important functions [3, 4].

Several studies in recent years have shown that circRNAs can function as miRNA sponges to sequester miRNAs [5–7]. It has also been reported that circRNAs are involved in regulation of transcription [8], neuronal development [9], cell cycle control [10], tumorigenesis, and chemoresistance [11, 12]. However, the functions of the majority circRNAs remain elusive.

Although some circRNAs are highly expressed in cells, the majority of circRNAs are low [13]. Therefore, the genetic approach of overexpressing circRNAs of interest will be a powerful tool to investigate their functions in various biological processes and contexts. It has been shown that *cis*-regulatory elements and

Christoph Dieterich and Argyris Papantonis (eds.), *Circular RNAs: Methods and Protocols*, Methods in Molecular Biology, vol. 1724, https://doi.org/10.1007/978-1-4939-7562-4_8, © Springer Science+Business Media, LLC 2018

trans-acting factors tightly regulate the biogenesis of circRNAs [13]; therefore, a few strategies have been employed to circularize RNAs using plasmid constructs [1, 5, 13, 14].

Firstly, complementary sequence-mediated RNA circularization is a classic strategy for circRNA overexpression [5, 10, 15]. Secondly, the insertion of RNA-binding motifs for Quaking into the introns flanking the desired exons facilitates the biogenesis of circRNAs [1]. In addition, a tRNA-based splicing mechanism was also employed to overexpress circRNAs [14]. However, there are a few drawbacks of these methods, such as low expression efficiency, inconvenience and length of time to make constructs, need for expression of RNA-binding protein in cells of interest, and inaccurate circRNA splicing which limits their application in circRNA functional analysis [5, 10, 14]. Therefore, there remains a need for a convenient, efficient, and accurate circRNA expression system.

To achieve this, we present a revision of the classic complementary sequence-mediated circRNA circularization for high-copy-number circRNA expression [5]. The circRNA expression cassette consists of three parts: two reverse complementary sequences (~800 bp of each) composed of the upstream intron of a particular gene (*MLLT3/AF9* for circR construct), and the circular RNA forming exons flanked by their specific upstream and downstream intronic sequences (~200 bp of each) to retain splicing recognition and polypyrimidine tracts (PPT). The upstream intron which is also inserted downstream of the circRNA exons generates a stable RNA hairpin structure after transcription which promotes exon splicing into circular RNA [5] (Fig. 1). By inserting the desired circRNA sequences into the MCS between the complementary intron sequences, the construct could be used as a generic construct for expressing various circRNAs of practically any sequence. Furthermore, our construct achieved higher circRNA expression than traditional cloning and 400–5000× higher than endogenous levels with high conversion efficiency exceeding 55%, minimizing by-products (Fig. 2). This strategy can be applied to amplify practically any circRNA, simplifying the cloning strategy in the process.

2   Materials

2.1 Construction of the circR Cloning Vector

1. The upstream intron fragment, the downstream intron fragment, and the desired circular RNA sequence.

2. The pcDNA3.1 His C plasmid (https://www.addgene.org/).

3. LB agar plate with 100 μg/mL ampicillin; LB broth with 100 μg/mL ampicillin.

4. High-fidelity DNA polymerase (Phusion, Thermo Fisher Scientific).

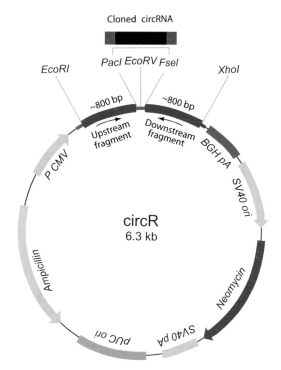

Fig. 1 The engineered circular RNA (circRNA) cassette consists of three parts: the upstream intron (~800 bp), the downstream intron fragment (the reverse complementary upstream intron sequence, ~800 bp), as well as the sequence for circRNA circularization which can be cloned in between the two complementary intron fragments (*PacI*, *EcoRV*, and *FseI* sites). The upstream intron fragment and the downstream fragment promote the circularization of the circRNA by back splicing. The inserted sequence for circRNA expression includes the circRNA forming sequence and its endogenous flanking genomic sequence which contains the splicing sites (~200 bp). The backbone of the circRNA expression construct is the pcDNA3.1 His C vector

5. Custom-designed oligonucleotide primers.
6. TAE (Tris–acetate–EDTA) buffer.
7. 1% Agarose gel.
8. T4 DNA ligase with 10× ligation buffer.
9. Restriction enzymes.
10. Chemically competent *Escherichia coli*.
11. PCR and gel purification kit.
12. Plasmid mini-prep kit.

2.2 Tissue Culture and Transfection

1. HEK 293T cell line.
2. DMEM medium (Dulbecco's modified Eagle medium, Thermo Fisher Scientific).
3. 10% Fetal calf serum (FCS).

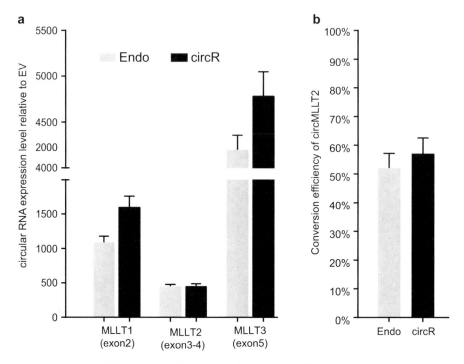

Fig. 2 Quantitative PCR (qPCR) analysis of *MLLT1*, *MLLT2*, and *MLLT3* circular RNA expression in different constructs. (**a**) The level of *MLLT1, MLLT2*, and *MLLT3* circular RNA expression in HEK 293T cells transfected with pcDNA3.1 construct (Endo) or circR construct overexpressing *circMLLT1*, *circ*MLLT2, and *circ*MLLT3, respectively. In the Endo constructs, the endogenous flanking sequence of each circular RNA sequence was used to promote its circular RNA circularization. Results were normalized to housekeeping gene *GAPDH* mRNA and each value shows the fold changes relative to the pcDNA3.1 empty vector samples. The error bar represents the standard error of the mean (SEM) of three independent experiments. (**b**) The conversion efficiency of *MLLT2* circular RNA from its expressed linear RNA in pcDNA3.1 (*MLLT2* Endo construct) and circR construct. The value was calculated by dividing the circular *MLLT2* by total *MLLT2* products (circular *MLLT2* ÷ linear *MLLT2*). The error bar represents the standard error of the mean (SEM) of three independent experiments

4. 1% Penicillin-streptomycin (10,000 U/mL, Thermo Fisher Scientific).

5. Tissue culture incubator.

6. Opti-MEM reduced serum media.

7. Lipofectamine reagent (LTX with Plus reagent, Invitrogen).

8. 12-Well tissue culture plate.

2.3 qPCR Validation of circRNA Expression

1. DEPC-treated water (Ambion).

2. TRIZOL Reagent (Invitrogen).

3. Ice-cold PBS.

4. Glycogen (5 mg/mL).

5. 70% ethanol.

6. 100% Isopropyl alcohol.

7. Chloroform.

8. NanoDrop machine.

9. QuantiTect reverse transcription kit (QIAGEN).

10. QuantiTect SYBR green kit (QIAGEN).

---

3 Methods

3.1 Construction of the circR Cloning Vector

Construction of the circR vectors was achieved by cloning the upstream and downstream intron fragments of *MLLT3/AF9* (**Note 1**) into the *Eco*RI/*Eco*RV and *Eco*RV/*Xho*I (reverse complement of above) sites of pcDNA3.1.

3.1.1 The Upstream Intron Cloning

1. PCR amplify the upstream intron sequence with appropriate genomic DNA template and PCR primers designed for restriction enzyme cloning, and check the PCR product by 1% agarose gel.

2. Digest the PCR product with appropriate restriction enzyme (EcoRI and EcoRV here), and purify the digested DNA with the ISOLATE II PCR and Gel Kit.

3. After EcoRI and EcoRV digestion of pcDNA3.1 His C plasmid, purify and recycle the digested linear plasmid by 1% agarose gel and the ISOLATE II PCR and Gel Kit.

4. Ligate the digested PCR product and plasmid by T4 ligase and transform the ligated products into chemically competent *E. coli* by heat shock.

5. Culture the transformed competent cells in LB medium supplemented with 100 μg/mL ampicillin at 37 °C, 200 rpm, overnight. Prepare plasmid after incubation by ISOLATE II plasmid mini Kit.

6. Digest the purified plasmid with appropriate restriction enzyme (*Eco*RI and *Eco*RV here), and check the DNA size on 1% agarose gel.

3.1.2 The Downstream Intron Cloning (the Inverted Upstream Intron Sequence) (*Note 2*)

1. PCR amplify the upstream intron sequence with appropriate genomic DNA template and PCR primers designed for restriction enzyme cloning, and check the PCR product by 1% agarose gel.

2. Digest the PCR product with appropriate restriction enzyme (EcoRV and XhoI here), and purify the digested DNA with the ISOLATE II PCR and Gel Kit.

3. After *Eco*RV and *Xho*I digestion of pcDNA3.1 His C plasmid containing the upstream intron fragment, purify and recycle the digested linear plasmid by 1% agarose gel and the ISOLATE II PCR and Gel Kit.

4. Ligate the digested PCR product and plasmid by T4 ligase and transform the ligated products into chemically competent *E. coli.*

5. Culture the transformed competent cells in LB medium supplemented with 100 μg/mL ampicillin at 37 °C, 200 rpm, overnight. Miniprep the culture to prepare plasmid after incubation.

6. Digest the purified plasmid with appropriate restriction enzyme (*Eco*RV and *Xho*I here), and check the DNA size on 1% agarose gel.

3.2 Inserting Desired Circular RNA Sequence (Includes the Endogenous Flanking Genomic Sequence ~200 bp Upstream and Downstream, Respectively)

The process of amplifying the circRNA exons and flanking splice recognition sites varies on whether the circRNA comprises a (1) single exon (monoexonic) or (2) multiple exons/intervening introns (Fig. 1). For a single exon only one PCR from gDNA is performed, with appropriate restriction enzyme overhangs. The forward primer is targeted to the intron immediately upstream of the exon (~200 bp upstream) and the reverse primer is ~200 bp downstream of the exon. This approach is also used for circRNAs with multiple exons and all intervening introns, amplifiable from genomic DNA alone. Compatible restriction enzyme sites are *Pac*I, *Fse*I, rare 8bp cutters, and *Eco*RV for blunt cloning.

To amplify the cassette for a multiple-exon circRNA (lacking intervening introns) requires three amplicons, followed by an overlapping PCR to fuse the three fragments. The first amplicon again starts upstream of first circRNA exon (~200 bp upstream) and incorporates some of the exon sequence (minimum 25 bp to allow overlap with the second fragment). The second fragment is exon specific, so it is amplified from cDNA starting at the first exon and ending with the terminal circRNA exon. The third fragment starts in the terminal exon (minimum 25 bp to allow sufficient overlap with the second fragment) and finishes ~200 bp downstream in the intron. A final overlap PCR where these three purified fragments are added as template and then amplified with the proximal and terminal primers is used in the first and third fragments with the PCR products subsequently cloned into the *Pac*I, *Eco*RV, or *Fse*I sites of the cloning vector.

1. PCR amplify the desired circular RNA sequence with appropriate cDNA and/or genomic DNA template and PCR primers designed for restriction enzyme cloning (possible restriction sites are *Pac*I, *Fse*I, rare 8bp cutters, or *Eco*RV for blunt cloning), and check the PCR product by 1% agarose gel.

2. Digest the PCR product with appropriate restriction enzyme (*Pac*I and *Eco*RV here), and purify the digested DNA with the ISOLATE II PCR and Gel Kit.

3. After *Pac*I and *Eco*RV digestion of pcDNA3.1 His C plasmid containing the upstream and downstream intron fragments,

purify and recycle the digested linear plasmid by 1% agarose gel and the ISOLATE II PCR and Gel Kit.

4. Ligate the digested PCR product and plasmid by T4 DNA ligase and transform the ligated products into chemically competent *E. coli*.

5. Culture the transformed competent cells in LB medium supplemented with 100 μg/mL ampicillin at 37 °C, 200 rpm, overnight. Miniprep the culture to prepare plasmid after incubation.

6. Digest the purified plasmid with appropriate restriction enzyme (*Pac*I and *Eco*RV here), and check the DNA size on 1% agarose gel.

7. Sanger sequencing to check the positive clones.

3.3 Tissue Culture and Transfection

Standard tissue culture and transfection protocols were applied in the experiment.

HEK293T cells are maintained in DMEM medium supplemented with 10% FCS and 1% penicillin/streptomycin at 37 °C, 5% CO_2. For cell passage, the cells were split 1:10 when the confluency reached approximately 80%.

1. The day before transfection, count and plate 2.5×10^5 cells per well in 1 mL of growth medium in a 12-well plate (no antibiotics).

2. On the day of transfection, for each well of cells, dilute 1 μg of plasmid DNA in 200 μL of Opti-MEM media, and then add 1 μL PLUS™ reagent (a 1:1 ratio to DNA) into the diluted DNA. Mix gently by pipetting up and down and then incubate at room temperature for 10 min.

3. For each well of cells, add 1.5 μL of Lipofectamine™ LTX into the above-diluted DNA solution (a 1:1.5 ratio to DNA). Mix gently by pipetting up and down and then incubate at room temperature for 25 min.

4. For each well of cells, add 200 μL of the above-mixed LTX-DNA complexes dropwise and mix gently by rocking the plate back and forth.

5. Incubate the cells for 48 h after transfection.

3.4 qPCR Validation of circRNA Expression

1. After 48-h transfection, remove media and rinse cells with ice-cold PBS once. Remove media and add 0.5 mL TriZol® (Thermo Fisher Scientific) to lyse cells directly in the tissue culture plate, and homogenize the samples by pipetting up and down a few times.

2. Incubate the homogenized samples at room temperature for 5 min, and then transfer each sample into 1.5 mL microfuge tubes.

3. Add 0.1 mL chloroform into each sample tube, vortex the samples vigorously for 15–30 s, and then incubate them at room temperature for 2–3 min.

4. Centrifuge the samples at 12,000 × g for 15 min at 4 °C, and then transfer the colorless upper aqueous phase to a new tube.

5. Add 0.25 mL isopropyl alcohol to precipitate RNA (**Note 3**), vortex and incubate the samples at room temperature for 10 min, then centrifuge the samples at 12,000 × g for 10 min at 4 °C, and discard the supernatant.

6. Wash the RNA pellet with 0.5 mL 75% ethanol, then centrifuge the samples at 7500 × g for 5 min at 4 °C, and remove the supernatant completely. Repeat above washing procedure once.

7. Air-dry the RNA pellet for 5–10 min (**Note 4**), then add 30 μL DEPC-treated water to dissolve RNA, and check the RNA quality on NanoDrop.

8. Reverse transcription from 1 μg total RNA performed with Quantiscript Reverse Transcriptase (Qiagen) according to the manufacturer's instructions, diluting 1:5 with MilliQ water.

9. Thaw Quantitect SYBR Green PCR kit (Qiagen) mastermix cDNA, and qPCR primers on ice. For each sample, prepare master mix for qPCR as follows (total volume 8 μL): 5 μL SYBR Green, 1 μL forward primer (10 μM), 1 μL reverse primer (10 μM), and 1 μL RNase-free water.

10. Dispense the master mix to PCR tubes, and add 2 μL of the cDNA into each PCR tube.

11. Run the qPCR as the protocol as follows: initial activation of HotStar Taq DNA polymerase for 15 min (at 95 °C), then followed by 45 cycles of denaturation (15 s at 94 °C), annealing (20 s at 60 °C), and extension (20 s at 72 °C).

4 Notes

1. The locus of the sequence is intron 4, chr9:20,414,651-20,415,428, hg38.

2. Cloning of the downstream intron fragment with the upstream intron fragment might lead to low yield of plasmid after mini-prep. If that happens, subclone the circRNA sequence before cloning the downstream intron fragment.

3. Add 1 μL glycogen (20 mg/mL) per sample to visualize RNA pellet after RNA precipitation.

4. Don't dry the RNA pellet completely as this will greatly decrease RNA solubility.

Acknowledgments

Research reported in this publication was supported by the National Health and Medical Research Council (NHMRC) project grant funding to S.J.C. (GNT1089167) and G.J.G. (GNT1089167, GNT1068773, GNT1126711). Fellowship support was provided by the Australian Research Council Future Fellowship to S.J.C. (FT160100318) and NHMRC Research Fellowship to G.J.G. (GNT1118170).

References

1. Conn SJ, Pillman KA, Toubia J, Conn VM, Salmanidis M et al (2015) The RNA binding protein quaking regulates formation of circRNAs. Cell 160:1125–1134

2. Jeck WR, Sharpless NE (2014) Detecting and characterizing circular RNAs. Nat Biotechnol 32:453–461

3. Rybak-Wolf A, Stottmeister C, Glazar P, Jens M, Pino N et al (2015) Circular RNAs in the mammalian brain are highly abundant, conserved, and dynamically expressed. Mol Cell 58:870–885

4. Jeck WR, Sorrentino JA, Wang K, Slevin MK, Burd CE et al (2013) Circular RNAs are abundant, conserved, and associated with ALU repeats. RNA 19:141–157

5. Hansen TB, Jensen TI, Clausen BH, Bramsen JB, Finsen B et al (2013) Natural RNA circles function as efficient microRNA sponges. Nature 495:384–388

6. Memczak S, Jens M, Elefsinioti A, Torti F, Krueger J et al (2013) Circular RNAs are a large class of animal RNAs with regulatory potency. Nature 495:333–338

7. Lasda E, Parker R (2014) Circular RNAs: diversity of form and function. RNA 20:1829–1842

8. Zhang Y, Zhang XO, Chen T, Xiang JF, Yin QF et al (2013) Circular intronic long noncoding RNAs. Mol Cell 51:792–806

9. You X, Vlatkovic I, Babic A, Will T, Epstein I et al (2015) Neural circular RNAs are derived from synaptic genes and regulated by development and plasticity. Nat Neurosci 18:603–610

10. Du WW, Yang W, Liu E, Yang Z, Dhaliwal P et al (2016) Foxo3 circular RNA retards cell cycle progression via forming ternary complexes with p21 and CDK2. Nucleic Acids Res 44:2846–2858

11. Guarnerio J, Bezzi M, Jeong JC, Paffenholz SV, Berry K et al (2016) Oncogenic role of fusion-circRNAs derived from cancer-associated chromosomal translocations. Cell 166:1055–1056

12. Yang W, Du WW, Li X, Yee AJ, Yang BB (2016) Foxo3 activity promoted by non-coding effects of circular RNA and Foxo3 pseudogene in the inhibition of tumor growth and angiogenesis. Oncogene 35:3919–3931

13. Chen LL (2016) The biogenesis and emerging roles of circular RNAs. Nat Rev Mol Cell Biol 17:205–211

14. Schmidt CA, Noto JJ, Filonov GS, Matera AG (2016) A method for expressing and imaging abundant, stable, circular RNAs in vivo using tRNA splicing. Methods Enzymol 572:215–236

15. Zhang XO, Wang HB, Zhang Y, Lu X, Chen LL et al (2014) Complementary sequence-mediated exon circularization. Cell 159:134–147

Chapter 9

Constructing GFP-Based Reporter to Study Back Splicing and Translation of Circular RNA

Yun Yang and Zefeng Wang

Abstract

Human transcriptome contains a large number of circular RNAs (circRNAs) that are mainly produced by back splicing of pre-mRNA. Here we describe a minigene reporter system containing a single exon encoding split GFP in reverse order, which can be efficiently back spliced to produce a circRNA encoding intact GFP gene. This simple reporter system can be adopted to study how different *cis*-elements and *trans*-factors affect circRNA production, and also can serve as a reliable system to measure the activity of IRES-mediated translation. Therefore this system can serve as a platform for mechanistic studies on the circRNA biogenesis and its function.

Key words Circular RNA, Back-splicing, Splicing reporter, Internal ribosomal entry sites, Cap-independent translation

1 Introduction

Most human genes undergo alternative splicing to produce multiple splicing isoforms with distinct activity, and the process of alternative splicing is tightly regulated by *cis*-regulatory elements and *trans*-acting splicing factors [1]. In a canonical splicing reaction, the splicing donor site (5′ splice site) is joined to a downstream splicing acceptor site (3′ splice site). However, splicing may sometimes happen in an unconventional back-splicing fashion where the splicing donor site can be joined to an upstream 3′ splice site, producing a circular RNA and a Y-shape intronic intermediate [2]. In addition to being promoted be intronic complementary sequences, the back splicing is probably also regulated by splicing factors that recognize *cis*-regulatory elements in pre-mRNA. However, the regulation of back splicing is not well understood.

The general functions of most circRNA remain unclear. An interesting possibility is that circRNAs may serve as mRNAs to direct protein synthesis, as the circRNAs containing internal ribosomal entry site (IRES) were found to be translated in vitro

Christoph Dieterich and Argyris Papantonis (eds.), *Circular RNAs: Methods and Protocols*, Methods in Molecular Biology, vol. 1724, https://doi.org/10.1007/978-1-4939-7562-4_9, © Springer Science+Business Media, LLC 2018

and in vivo [3, 4]. To study the regulation of circRNA production, we developed a single exon that can be efficiently back spliced to generate circRNA. The resulting circRNA can be translated from an IRES to generate a functional GFP protein. Using this simple reporter, we have made several fundamental discoveries related to the biogenesis and function of circRNA. For example, we found that the back splicing is enhanced by intronic complementary sequences that form double-stranded RNA (dsRNA) structure, but such structure is not required. Moreover, back splicing is regulated by general splicing factors and *cis*-elements, but with regulatory rules distinct from canonical splicing [4]. Surprisingly, we found that many sites contain *N-6-methyladenosine* that can efficiently drive protein translation from this circRNA reporter, and such translation from circRNA is promoted by cellular stress [5].

2   Materials

Prepare all solutions using ultrapure water and analytical grade reagents (unless indicated otherwise). Prepare and store all reagents at room temperature (unless indicated otherwise). Diligently follow all waste disposal regulations when disposing waste materials.

2.1   Plasmid Construction

1. pEGFP-C1 and pIRES2-EGFP: Purchase from Takara Bio USA, Mountain View, CA, USA. pGZ3 vector was previously constructed as a modular splicing reporter [6, 7]. All vectors were stored at −20 °C.

2. Restriction enzymes (*Age*I, *Bam*HI, *Bgl*II, *Sal*I, *Xba*I, *Xho*I): Purchase from New England Biolabs, Ipswich, MA, USA. Store at −20 °C.

3. Phusion® high-fidelity DNA polymerase: Purchase from New England Biolabs, Ipswich, MA, USA. Store at −20 °C.

4. T4 DNA ligase (1 U/μL): Purchase from Thermo Fisher Scientific, Grand Island, NY, USA. Store at −20 °C.

5. QIAquick PCR purification kit and Gel extraction kit: Purchase from Qiagen, Germantown, MD, USA.

6. Agarose: Purchase from Thermo Fisher Scientific, Grand Island, NY, USA.

7. Ethidium bromide solution (10 mg/mL): Purchase from BIO-RAD, Hercules, CA, USA.

8. 50× TAE electrophoresis buffer: 2 M Tris, 1 M acetic acid, 50 mM EDTA. Dilute 50× TAE electrophoresis buffer to 1× TAE electrophoresis buffer before use.

9. Subcloning Efficiency™ DH5α™ Competent Cells: Purchase from Thermo Fisher Scientific, Grand Island, NY, USA.

10. LB broth with kanamycin: 1.0% Tryptone, 0.5% yeast extract, 1.0% NaCl, 50 μg/mL kanamycin.

11. QIAprep spin miniprep kit: Purchase from Qiagen, Germantown, MD, USA.

2.2 Cell Culture

1. DMEM medium–high glucose: Purchase from Thermo Fisher Scientific, Grand Island, NY, USA. Store at 4 °C.

2. Fetal bovine serum: Purchase from Thermo Fisher Scientific, Grand Island, NY, USA. Store at −20 °C.

3. DMEM with 10% FBS: Add 50 mL FBS to 450 mL DMEM medium–high glucose and mix by pipetting. Store at 4 °C.

4. Trypsin–EDTA (0.05%), phenol red: Purchase from Thermo Fisher Scientific, Grand Island, NY, USA. Store at 4 °C.

5. Lipofectamine® 2000 transfection reagent: Purchase from Thermo Fisher Scientific, Grand Island, NY, USA. Store at 4 °C.

6. Opti-MEM® I reduced-serum medium: Purchase from Thermo Fisher Scientific, Grand Island, NY, USA. Store at 4 °C.

7. 1× PBS buffer: Purchase from Thermo Fisher Scientific, Grand Island, NY, USA. Store at 4 °C.

2.3 Reverse Transcription and PCR

1. TRIzol® reagent: Purchase from Thermo Fisher Scientific, Grand Island, NY, USA. Store at 4 °C.

2. TURBO DNA-*free*™ kit: Purchase from Thermo Fisher Scientific, Grand Island, NY, USA. Store at −20 °C.

3. RNase R: Purchase from Epicentre, Madison, WI, USA. Store at −20 °C.

4. SuperScript® III first-strand synthesis system: Purchase from Thermo Fisher Scientific, Grand Island, NY, USA. Store at −20 °C.

5. One*Taq*® DNA polymerase: Purchase from New England Biolabs, Ipswich, MA, USA. Store at −20 °C.

6. Deoxynucleotide (dNTP) solution mix (10 mM): Purchase from New England Biolabs, Ipswich, MA, USA. Store at −20 °C.

2.4 SDS Polyacrylamide Gel

1. 1.5 M Tris–HCl (pH 8.8, to prepare resolving gel): Dissolve 181.5 g Tris base in 900 mL ultrapure water. Adjust pH to 8.8 using HCl. Make up to 1 L with water.

2. 0.5 M Tris–HCl (pH 6.8, to prepare stacking gel): Dissolve 60 g Tris base in 900 mL ultrapure water. Adjust pH to 6.8 using HCl. Make up to 1 L with water.

3. 40% Acrylamide/Bis solution (37.5:1): Purchase from AMRESCO, Solon, OH, USA. Store at 4 °C.

4. Ammonium persulfate: Purchase from SIGMA-ALDRICH, St. Louis, MO. Make 10% solution in water before use (*see* **Note 1**).

5. *N,N,N′,N′*-Tetramethylethylenediamine (TEMED): Purchase from SIGMA-ALDRICH, St. Louis, MO, USA.

6. SDS-PAGE running buffer: 25 mM Tris–HCl, pH 8.3, 0.192 M glycine, 0.1% SDS.

7. RIPA buffer: 25 mM Tris–HCl pH 7.6, 150 mM NaCl, 1% NP-40, 1% sodium deoxycholate, 0.1% SDS. Purchase from Thermo Fisher Scientific, Grand Island, NY, USA. Store at 4 °C. Before use, add cOmplete™, EDTA-free Protease Inhibitor Cocktail (purchase from SIGMA-ALDRICH, St. Louis, MO, USA) (*see* **Note 2**).

8. 2× Laemmli loading buffer: 65.8 M Tris–HCl, pH 6.8, 26.3% glycerol, 2.1% SDS, 0.01% bromophenol blue. Purchase from BIO-RAD, Hercules, CA, USA. Add 50 μL of 2-mercaptoethanol per 950 μL before use (*see* **Note 3**).

9. Mini-PROTEAN® Tetra Handcast Systems: Purchase from BIO-RAD, Hercules, CA, USA.

10. Prestained protein standard—dual color: Purchase from BIO-RAD, Hercules, CA, USA. Store at −20 °C.

2.5 Immunoblotting and Flow Cytometry

1. Immun-Blot® PVDF membranes. Purchase from BIO-RAD, Hercules, CA, USA.

2. Towbin transfer buffer: 25 mM Tris–HCl, pH 8.3, 0.192 M glycine, 20% methanol.

3. Tris-buffered saline with Tween-20 (TBST, 10×): 1.5 M NaCl, 0.1 M Tris–HCl, pH 7.4, 0.5% Tween-20.

4. Membrane-blocking solution and antibody diluent solution: 5% Milk in TBST. Store at 4 °C (*see* **Note 4**).

5. Blot absorbent filter paper: Purchase from BIO-RAD, Hercules, CA, USA.

6. GFP antibody (632381): Purchase from Takara Bio USA, Mountain View, CA, USA. Store at −20 °C. GAPDH antibody (sc-47724): Purchase from Santa Cruz Biotechnology, Dallas, TX, USA. Goat anti-mouse IgG-HRP (sc-2005): Purchase from Santa Cruz Biotechnology, Dallas, TX, USA. Store at 4 °C.

7. Amersham ECL Prime Western Blotting Detection Reagent: Purchase from GE Healthcare Life Sciences, Pittsburgh, PA, USA. Store at 4 °C.

8. Propidium iodide (PI, 1 mg/mL): Purchase from Thermo Fisher Scientific, Grand Island, NY, USA.

9. PI staining solution: 100 μg/mL PI in PBS stored at 4 °C in the dark.

10. FACS™ tubes (5 mL round-bottom polystyrene tubes): Purchase from Thermo Fisher Scientific, Grand Island, NY, USA.

3 Methods

Carry out all procedures at room temperature unless otherwise specified.

3.1 Plasmid Construction

1. An IRES-G (IRES and N-terminal GFP sequences) fragment is amplified by Phusion high-fidelity DNA polymerase (PCR reaction and condition setup as in Tables 1 and 2) using pIRES2-EGFP as templates with primers (primers 1 and 2 in Table 3) containing *Bgl*II/*Xho*I restriction sites.

2. PCR product is purified by QIAquick PCR purification kit according to the manufacture's protocol.

3. IRES-G fragment is digested with *Bgl*II and *Xho*I, and pEGFP-C1 is digested with *Bgl*II and *Sal*I in 6 h at 37 °C (*see* **Note 5**).

4. Load digested fragment and plasmid into 1% agarose gel with 0.5 μg/mL ethidium bromide, and electrophorese at 100 V for 40 min.

5. Cut the digested fragment and plasmid band from the gel, and extract DNA using QIAquick gel extraction kit according to the manufacturer's protocol.

6. Ligate IRES-G fragment (*Bgl*II/*Xho*I) into pEGFP-C1 (*Bgl*II/*Sal*I) using T4 DNA ligase at 16 °C in 1 h.

Table 1
PCR reaction setup (Phusion high-fidelity DNA polymerase)

Component	50 μL reaction
Nuclease-free water	to 50 μL
5× Phusion HF buffer	10 μL
10 mM dNTPs	1 μL
10 μM forward primer	2.5 μL
10 μM reverse primer	2.5 μL
Template DNA	1 ng plasmid
Phusion DNA polymerase	0.5 μL

Table 2
Thermocycling conditions (Phusion high-fidelity DNA polymerase)

Step	Temperature (°C)	Time
Initial denaturation	98	30 s
25–35 cycles	98	10 s
	58	20 s
	72	30 s
Final extension	72	5 min
Hold	4–10	

7. Transform the ligation product (called pCIRC-IRES-G) into DH5α competent cells according to the manufacturer's protocol.

8. Pick clones into LB with kanamycin and incubate at 37 °C for 10 h.

9. Isolate plasmid by QIAprep spin miniprep kit according to the manufacturer's protocol and sequence plasmid using Sanger sequencing.

10. An intron-FP (intron 12 of IGF2BP1 and C-terminal GFP sequences) fragment is amplified by Phusion high-fidelity DNA polymerase (PCR reaction and condition setup as in Tables 1 and 2) using pGZ3 vector as templates with primers (primers 3 and 4 in Table 3) containing AgeI/BamHI sites, and then inserted into pCIRC-IRES-G that was cut with AgeI/BglII, named pCIRC-FP-IRES-G.

11. To generate the structured intron circular RNA reporter, the reverse complementary fragment of partial intron 12 of IGF2BP1 was amplified using pGZ3 vector as templates with primers (primers 5 and 6 in Table 3) containing XbaI/BamHI sites, and subsequently inserted into pCIRC-FP-IRES-G that was digested with BamHI/XbaI. To generate the unstructured intron circular RNA reporter, the part of intron 12 of IGF2BP1 was amplified using pGZ3 vector as templates with primers (primers 7 and 8 in Table 3) containing BamHI/XbaI sites, and subsequently inserted into pCIRC-FP-IRES-G that was digested with BamHI/XbaI.

3.2 Cell Culture and Transfection

1. HEK293 cells are cultured with DMEM medium containing 10% of FBS at 37 °C and 5% CO_2.

2. To transiently express circRNA reporter, HEK293 cells are plated into 12-well plates 1 day before transfection.

3. Plasmids (1 μg/per well) were transfected into HEK293 cells using Lipofectamine 2000 according to the manufacturer's manual (*see* **Note 6**).

Table 3
List of oligonucleotide sequences used in this study

Primer #	Name	Sequence	Notes
1	IRES-G-Fwd	TCACAGATCTGAATTCTGCAGTCGA CGATCCGCCCCTCTCCCTCC	Used to clone IRES-G region into pEGFP-C1 vector
2	GFP-E1-R	CACCTCGAGACTTACCTGGACGTAG CCTTCGG	
3	pGZ3-Int2-F	CACACCGGTGACTGAACATGGAGG AATTG	Used for cloning intron-FP region into pEGFP-C1 vector
4	GFP-E2-R-new	CACGGATCCTTACTTGTACAGCTC GTCCATG	
5	Xba-intron-fwd	CACTCTAGAAGAGGCCCAATTCAA GGATTTGG	Used for cloning structured intron into the minigene
6	BamHI-intron-rev	CACGGATCCCAAATAAGATGCCCTCAGAC	
7	Xba-intron-rev	TCTAGAAGAGGCCCAATTCAAGGATTTGG	Used for cloning unstructured intron into the minigene
8	BamHI-intron-fwd	CACGGATCCCAAATAAGATGCCCTCAGAC	
9	Gexon1f	AGTGCTTCAGCCGCTACCC	Used for detecting circular GFP
10	Gexon3r	GTTGTACTCCAGCTTGTGCC	
11	Linear-F	ACGTAAACGGCCACAAGTTC	Used for detecting linear GFP
12	Linear-R	CTGAGGGCATCTTATTTGGG	

4. Incubate the cells at 37 °C for 48 h.

5. Dissociate cells by trypsin–EDTA at 37 °C for 2 min. Inactive trypsin by adding 2× volume of DMEM medium containing 10% of FBS.

6. Pipet dissociated cells into 1.5 mL tube, and centrifuge at 2000 rpm (400 × g) for 2 min.

7. Remove the supernatant and wash the cell pellet by PBS. Store the cell pellet at −80 °C.

3.3 Reverse Transcription and PCR

1. Isolate total RNA by TRIzol reagent according to the manufacturer's instructions (see **Note 7**).

2. To remove genomic DNA, treat total RNA with DNase I using TURBO DNA-*free*™ kit according to the manufacturer's instructions.

3. Incubate total RNA (1 μg) with or without RNase R at 37 °C for 2 h.

4. Treated RNAs are reverse-transcribed with SuperScript III with random priming according to the manufacturer's manual.

5. Circular and linear GFP fragments are amplified by One$Taq^{®}$ DNA polymerase (PCR reaction and condition setup as in Tables 4 and 5) using RT products as templates with primers (primers 11 and 12 or 13 and 14 in Table 3).

6. Load digested fragment and plasmid into 1.5% agarose gel with 0.5 μg/mL ethidium bromide, and electrophorese at 100 V for 40 min (*see* **Note 8**).

7. Image the gel by Bio-Rad ChemiDoc Imaging Systems (*see* Fig. 1).

3.4 Western Blot

1. Add 50 μL ice-cold RIPA buffer with protease inhibitor to samples (50 μL lysis buffer per well sample).

2. Incubate on ice for 20 min, and centrifuge at 12,000 rpm ($14,000 \times g$), 4 °C, for 20 min.

3. Aspirate the supernatant and place in a fresh tube kept on ice, and discard the pellet.

Table 4
PCR reaction setup (One$Taq^{®}$ DNA polymerase)

Component	25 μL reaction
Nuclease-free water	to 25
5× OneTaq standard reaction buffer	5
10 mM dNTPs	0.5
10 μM Forward primer	0.5
10 μM Reverse primer	0.5
cDNA	1
OneTaq DNA polymerase	0.125

Table 5
Thermocycling conditions (One$Taq^{®}$ DNA polymerase)

Step	Temperature (°C)	Time
Initial denaturation	94	30 s
22 cycles	94	20 s
	58	25 s
	68	25 s
Final extension	68	5 min
Hold	4	

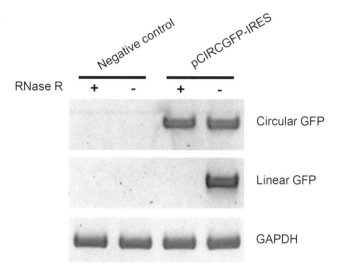

Fig. 1 Detection of circular GFP RNA expression from pCIRCGFP-IRES by RT-PCR with RNase R treatment. HEK 293 cells transiently transfected with control and pCIRCGFP-IRES plasmid are collected at 48 h after transfection. Total RNAs are purified using TRIzol, treated with or without RNase R, and analyzed by semi-quantitative RT-PCRs using various primer sets

4. Add 50 μL 2× Laemmli sample buffer into supernatant, and boil samples at 95 °C for 5 min.

5. Load 20 μL samples into wells of 10% SDS-PAGE gel, and run the gel at 100 V till the dye front reaches the bottom of the gel (*see* **Note 9**).

6. Activate PVDF membrane with methanol for 2 min and put the membrane into transfer buffer.

7. Rinse the SDS-PAGE gel with transfer buffer, and set up "transfer sandwich" (cathode(−)—pad—filter paper—gel—PVDF membrane—filter paper—pad—anode(+)).

8. Transfer protein from the gel to membrane at 75 V 4 °C for 75 min (*see* **Note 10**).

9. Block the PVDF membrane for 1 h at room temperature using blocking buffer.

10. Wash the PVDF membrane once by TBST, and incubate the membrane with GFP antibody (1:2000 dilution) or GAPDH antibody (1:3000 dilution) at 4 °C overnight (*see* **Note 11**).

11. Wash the membrane by TBST three times, 5 min each.

12. Incubate the membrane with goat anti-mouse IgG-HRP antibody (1:5000 dilution) for 1 h at room temperature.

13. Wash the membrane by TBST three times, 5 min each.

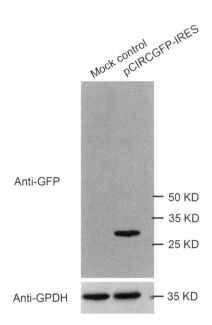

Fig. 2 Detection of GFP protein expression from pCIRCGFP-IRES by western blot. HEK 293 cells transiently transfected with control and pCIRCGFP-IRES plasmid are assayed by western blot at 48 h after transfection

14. Develop the signal by Amersham ECL Prime Western Blotting Detection Reagent (following the manufacturer's instructions).

15. Acquire images by Bio-Rad ChemiDoc Imaging Systems (see Fig. 2).

3.5 Flow Cytometry

1. Dissociate cells by trypsin–EDTA at 37 °C for 2 min after 48-h transfection.

2. Inactive trypsin by adding 2× volumes of DMEM medium containing 10% of FBS.

3. Pipet dissociated cells into FACS™ tubes, and centrifuge at 300 × g for 5 min.

4. Remove the supernatant and wash the cell pellet by 1 mL PBS twice.

5. Resuspend cells in 200 μL of PBS (*see* **Note 12**).

6. Add 4 μL of PI staining solution into samples. Mix gently and incubate for 5 min in the dark.

7. Acquire data by FACSCalibur fluorescence-activated cell sorter (FACS) or other similar analyzer (*see* Fig. 3).

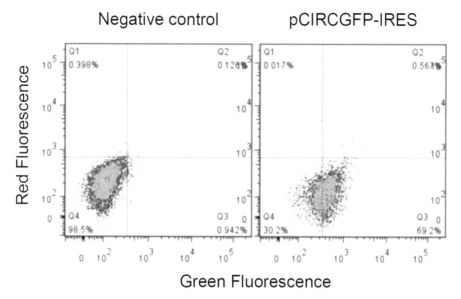

Fig. 3 Detection of GFP protein expression from pCIRCGFP-IRES by flow cytometry. HEK 293 cells transiently transfected with mock control and pCIRCGFP-IRES plasmid are assayed by flow cytometry at 48 h after transfection

4   Notes

1. It is best to make this fresh each time.

2. To make 25× stock solution, dissolve one cOmplete EDTA-free tablet in 2 mL water or in 2 mL PBS buffer, pH 7.0. The stock solution can be stored at 4 °C for 2 weeks, or at −20 °C for 2 months.

3. It is best to make this fresh each time.

4. To prevent microbial contamination, sodium azide can be added to blocking buffer and dilution buffer to a final concentration of 0.02% (w/v). Diluted antibodies can be reused 2–3 times in 1 week (store at 4 °C).

5. To prevent plasmid self-ligation, digested plasmid can be dephosphorylated by shrimp alkaline phosphatase (rSAP). After digestion, inactive the restriction enzyme by heating at 80 °C for 20 min. Then, add 1 U rSAP to solution and incubate at 37 °C for 30 min. Finally, inactive rSAP by heating at 65 °C for 5 min and purify the digested vector by gel purification.

6. Prepare DNA-lipid complexes using a DNA (μg) to Lipofectamine® 2000 (μL) ratio of 1:2 for HEK293 cells.

7. For RNA extraction and RT-PCR experiments, use nuclease-free tubes, tips, and reagents.

8. To get a good gel figure, we suggest to run a DNA polyacrylamide gel (6–8%).

9. Usually, it will take 2 h. If you want to run a gel as fast as possible, it can run at 200 V 4 °C. It may take 35–45 min. If you want to get sharp bands, you can run the gel at 65 V for 30 min and change the voltage to 100 V.

10. Transfer at 30 V overnight in the cold room will help the transfer of high-molecular-weight protein.

11. Blocked membranes can also be incubated with primary antibody at room temperature for 1–2 h.

12. It is best to filter your samples before running on any cytometer. You can use commercial filters (e.g., Falcon cell strainers) or bulk nylon mesh filter (e.g., Millipore nylon net filter).

References

1. Wang Z, Burge CB (2008) Splicing regulation: from a parts list of regulatory elements to an integrated splicing code. RNA 14:802–813. https://doi.org/10.1261/rna.876308

2. Chen LL (2016) The biogenesis and emerging roles of circular RNAs. Nat Rev Mol Cell Biol 17:205–211. https://doi.org/10.1038/nrm.2015.32

3. Chen CY, Sarnow P (1995) Initiation of protein synthesis by the eukaryotic translational apparatus on circular RNAs. Science 268:415–417

4. Wang Y, Wang Z (2015) Efficient backsplicing produces translatable circular mRNAs. RNA 21:172–179. https://doi.org/10.1261/rna.048272.114

5. Yang Y, Fan X, Mao M, Song X, Wu P, Jin Y, Yang Y, Wong C, Xiao X, Wang Z (2017) Extensive translation of circular RNAs driven by N6-methyladenosine. Cell Res 27:626–641

6. Wang Y, Ma M, Xiao X, Wang Z (2012) Intronic splicing enhancers, cognate splicing factors and context-dependent regulation rules. Nat Struct Mol Biol 19:1044–1052. https://doi.org/10.1038/nsmb.2377

7. Wang Y, Wang Z (2014) Systematical identification of splicing regulatory cis-elements and cognate trans-factors. Methods 65:350–358. https://doi.org/10.1016/j.ymeth.2013.08.019

Chapter 10

Northern Blot Analysis of Circular RNAs

Tim Schneider, Silke Schreiner, Christian Preußer, Albrecht Bindereif, and Oliver Rossbach

Abstract

Northern blotting enables the specific detection and characterization of RNA molecules. Recently, circular RNAs (circRNAs) were described as a new class of cell type-specific noncoding RNAs. With the discovery of many novel circRNAs on the basis of high-throughput sequencing and bioinformatics, a solid biochemical approach is required to directly detect and validate specific circRNA species. Here we give a detailed overview of how different Northern blot methods can be employed to validate specific circRNAs. Different Northern gel and detection systems are introduced, in combination with additional tools for circRNA characterization, such as RNase R and RNase H treatments.

Key words Northern blot, Circular RNA, circRNA, Denaturing glyoxal agarose gel, Northern transfer, Digoxigenin-detection system, Riboprobes, Junction probes, RNase R, RNase H

1 Introduction

Circular RNAs (circRNAs) have within the last few years emerged as a new class on noncoding RNAs that are widespread in all eukaryotes analyzed so far [1, 2]. Historically, circRNAs date back to the 1970s, when viroid RNAs, powerful plant pathogens, had been identified as the first circRNA species [3]. However, only in 2012/2013 systematic sequencing-based approaches uncovered circRNAs as a large new class of noncoding RNA [4–6]. Functionally, except for miRNA sponging [6, 7], circRNAs are still largely unexplored, which presents a great challenge for the next decade.

Based on initial studies on circRNA biogenesis and on RNA-Seq analyses, most circRNAs are exonic and derived from precursors of protein-coding mRNAs (pre-mRNAs), whereby one exon or several adjacent, spliced exons are excised in circular configuration, based on a kind of alternative splicing mechanism sometimes called "back splicing" ([8], and references therein).

Christoph Dieterich and Argyris Papantonis (eds.), *Circular RNAs: Methods and Protocols*, Methods in Molecular Biology, vol. 1724, https://doi.org/10.1007/978-1-4939-7562-4_10, © Springer Science+Business Media, LLC 2018

Because of this very young history of circRNAs as a novel RNA class, there is some uncertainty about the necessary standards and stringent quality criteria: What is essential to establish a newly discovered RNA species as circRNA? After initial bioinformatic search and circRNA identification, usually based on the characteristic circular splice junction, experimental validation approaches are important: For that, RT-PCR assays and Northern blotting have become the standard approaches. This chapter concentrates on Northern blot analysis of circRNAs, which still represents a gold standard for circRNA validation and characterization.

For appreciating the value of Northern blot hybridization in circRNA analysis, we have to point out the limitations of RT-PCR assays. RT-PCR provides initial experimental evidence for circularity and an easy and rapid means for circRNA detection: Primer pairs flanking the circular splice site [divergent relative to the circularizing exon(s)] are designed to generate a suitable PCR product (usually 100–200 nt).

However, linear *trans*-spliced RNA isoforms may generate the same RT-PCR products as putative circRNAs. Therefore, to unequivocally prove circularity requires more than RT-PCR. One possibility is to combine RT-PCR assays with prior RNase R treatment (*see* below under Subheading 3.7). RNase R is an exoribonuclease, and most circRNAs are resistant, in contrast to linear RNA species, which can be degraded by RNase R. Unfortunately, there are limitations in the validity of RNase R assays, since-on the one hand-relatively large circRNAs tend to be not absolutely RNase R resistant; on the other hand, stable structures in linear RNAs may also block RNase R digestion. In sum, although RT-PCR assays in combination with RNase R digests can be done in medium-throughput scale, and can be quantitated by real-time PCR, they do not yield definitive biochemical proof for circularity.

The second approach is Northern blot hybridization, which represents the method of choice to convincingly demonstrate circular configuration of putative circRNAs. Specific circRNA detection can be accomplished by short probes spanning the circular splice junction, or by longer probes covering as much as an entire circularized exon. This latter option becomes relevant if specificity for the circular isoform is not essential (for example, if the linear forms do not enter the gel, or if both linear and circular isoforms should be detected in parallel, or in case of exclusively circular RNAs).

Although somewhat more laborious and time consuming, Northern blots are therefore essential parts of any circRNA characterization, due to their great versatility. First, the choice of probe regions (circular or linear splice junction or exonic regions, Subheading 3.4) and detection principle (digoxigenin [DIG] or ^{32}P-labeled probes, Subheadings 3.5 or 3.6) determines the specificity for circular versus linear isoforms. Second, the choice of the gel matrix adds more flexibility in Northern blot assays. For example, circular and linear RNA species exhibit size-dependent characteristics in their electrophoretic behavior (glyoxal agarose/denaturing polyacrylamide; percentage agarose/polyacrylamide). Agarose gels are suitable for circRNAs from 0.2 kb up to several kb. Note that in agarose gels, circular and linear RNAs of the same size cannot be distinguished by their running behavior. On the contrary, in denaturing polyacrylamide gels, linear RNA runs at the expected size, whereas circRNAs have a lower apparent mobility relative to linear markers; this retardation effect is enhanced by increasing acrylamide concentrations [9]. Due to this limitation, circRNAs only up to 1 kb can be analyzed by polyacrylamide gel electrophoresis.

Therefore, at least for a comprehensive analysis of one or a few putative circRNAs, not for a medium- to high-throughput screening efforts, Northern blot assays provide a very valuable and highly informative approach.

2   Materials

All solutions should be prepared with deionized and ultrapure water (e.g., Milli-Q system). Prepare and store all solutions at room temperature (unless indicated otherwise). Some solutions can be used for both glyoxal agarose and denaturing polyacrylamide Northern blotting.

2.1   Glyoxal Agarose Gel

1. 10× MOPS agarose running buffer (stock and working solution): 10× Stock solution of 200 mM 3-(N-morpholino) propanesulfonic acid (MOPS), 50 mM sodium acetate, 10 mM EDTA (pH 8.0), pH to be adjusted to 7.0 using NaOH. This solution is used for preparation of a 1× buffer for agarose electrophoresis.

2. ddH$_2$O treated with 0.1% dimethyl pyrocarbonate (DMPC; stir for 1 h, autoclaved twice).

3. 1.2% Agarose in 1× MOPS running buffer.

4. Glyoxal sample buffer: NorthernMax-Gly Sample Loading Dye (contains ethidium bromide, Thermo Fisher).

5. RNA ladder (0.2–6 kb, RiboRuler high range, Thermo Fisher).

6. DIG-labeled DNA molecular weight marker VII (0.35–8.5 kb, Roche).

7. Heat block capable of heating up to 95 °C.

2.2   Denaturing Polyacrylamide Gel

1. 10× TBE running and blotting buffer: 10× Stock solution of 890 mM H$_3$BO$_3$, 890 mM Tris, and 20 mM EDTA (pH 8.0). This solution is used for gel preparation of a 1× buffer for electrophoresis and blotting.

2. ddH$_2$O treated with 0.1% DMPC (stir for 1 h, autoclave twice).

3. 6% Acrylamide/bis-acrylamide (stock solution: 40% 19:1, Roth) in 1× TBE, 50% (w/v) urea.

4. 10% Ammonium peroxodisulfate (APS).

5. *N, N, N′, N′*-tetramethyl-ethylenediamine (TEMED).

6. 2× Formamide loading buffer: 90% deionized formamide, 1× TBE, 0.05% (w/v) bromophenol blue, 0.05% (w/v) xylene cyanol.

7. DIG-labeled DNA molecular weight marker VIII (0.02–1.1 kb, Roche).

8. Heat block capable of heating up to 95 °C.

2.3 Electroblotting

1. 1× TBE blotting buffer: 89 mM H$_3$BO$_3$, 89 mM Tris, and 2 mM EDTA (pH 8.0).

2. Tris–HCl: 50 mM Tris, pH adjusted to 8.0 with HCl (only for glyoxal agarose Northern blot).

3. Semidry electrophoretic transfer cell: Trans-Blot Semi-Dry Transfer System (Biorad).

4. Blotting paper: Thick blot filter paper (7.5 × 10 cm or 15 × 20 cm, Biorad).

5. Nylon blotting membrane (Hybond-N+, GE Healthcare).

6. Crosslinker: BLX-254 (Bio-Link).

7. Plastic containers.

2.4 DIG-Detection System

1. NorthernMax hybridization buffer (Thermo Fisher): 20× SSC washing buffer (stock and working solution): 3 M NaCl, 300 mM sodium citrate, pH to be adjusted to 7.0 using HCl. Autoclave for storage. This buffer is used for preparation of 2× and 0.5× washing buffers supplemented with 0.1% (w/v) SDS.

2. Maleic acid (stock and working solution): 1 M Maleic acid stock solution, pH to be adjusted to 7.5 using NaOH. Autoclave for storage. This solution is used for the preparation of a 100 mM maleic acid buffer by 1:10 dilution.

3. DIG washing buffer: Maleic acid buffer (100 mM, pH 7.5) supplemented with 0.3% (v/v) Tween-20.

4. DIG-blocking solution: 2% (w/v) blocking reagent (Roche) in maleic acid buffer (100 mM, pH 7.5, *see* **Note 1**).

5. DIG-detection buffer: 100 mM Tris, 100 mM NaCl, pH adjusted to 9.5 with HCl.

6. For DIG-labeled riboprobes: DIG RNA labeling mix (Roche), HiScribe T7 High Yield RNA Synthesis Kit (NEB), mini Quick Spin RNA Columns (Roche).

7. Hybridization oven and tubes: 35 × 150/300 mm hybridization tubes.

8. Anti-DIG antibody: Fab-fragment coupled to alkaline phosphatase (Roche).

9. DIG-detection substrate: CPD-star (Roche).

10. Saran foil.

11. X-ray films: Amersham Hyperfilm ECL (18 × 24 cm, GE Healthcare), film cassette.

12. Processing machine: AGFA Curix 60 tabletop processor.

2.5 Detection by ^{32}P-Radiolabeled Oligonucleotides

1. Single-stranded oligonucleotides of 20–30 nt in length with 5'-hydroxyl group (*see* **Note 2**).

2. [γ-^{32}P]-ATP.

3. T4 polynucleotide kinase (NEB).

4. Mini Quick Spin Oligo Columns (Roche).

5. ULTRAhyb Ultrasensitive Hybridization Buffer (Thermo Fisher).

6. 20× SSC washing buffer (stock and working solution): 3 M NaCl, 300 mM sodium citrate, pH to be adjusted to 7.0 using HCl. Autoclave for storage. This buffer is used for preparation of 2× and 0.1× washing buffers supplemented with 0.1% (w/v) SDS.

7. X-ray films suitable for autoradiography or phosphor imaging screens.

8. Film cassette (with intensifier screen if X-ray films are used).

3 Methods

3.1 Agarose Gel Electrophoresis of RNA

1. Prepare 50 mL of 1.2% agarose in 1× MOPS buffer (without ethidium bromide, *see* **Note 3**) and cast a thin gel with the following dimensions: 11 × 9 × 0.5 cm (=50 mL, *see* **Note 4**). Allow to cool for 30 min.

2. Add glyoxal loading buffer (contains ethidium bromide) 1:1 to the RNA samples (1–50 μg total RNA in 10 μL DMPC-H_2O) as well as the RNA (2 μL) and DIG-labeled DNA ladder (2 μL, DIG VII). Incubate for 30 min at 50 °C, briefly spin down, and place on ice (*see* Fig. 1a, **Note 5**).

3. Load the denatured RNA samples and size markers onto the gel and electrophorese for 1–2 h (depending on the target RNA size) at 100 V. After the run is completed, image the gel by UV documentation of ethidium bromide staining (size markers and ribosomal RNAs should be visible, *see* **Note 6**).

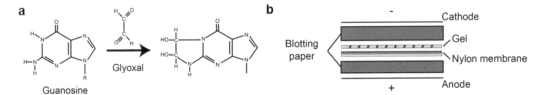

Fig. 1 Reaction of guanosine residues in RNA with glyoxal and blot assembly for membrane transfer of RNA. (**a**) The covalent adduct prevents normal base pairing and maintains the RNA in a denatured state in agarose gels. Once formed, these adducts are stable at room temperature at pH <7.0 [13]. (**b**) Schematic representation of an assembled transfer sandwich used for glyoxal agarose and denaturing polyacrylamide Northern blotting

4. Prior to electroblotting, equilibrate the gel in 1× TBE blotting buffer for 20 min. For further reading on agarose gel electrophoresis of RNA, *see* also ref. [10–12].

3.2 Denaturing Polyacrylamide Gel Electrophoresis of RNA

1. Clean two glass plates with H_2O and ethanol; make sure that they are dry and fat free. Assemble the plates with spacers and fix them with metal clamps. The gel is cast in horizontal position (*see* **Note 7**).

2. Prepare 30 mL of a 6% acrylamide/bis-acrylamide mix (19:1, in 1× TBE) with 50% (w/v) urea. For polymerization first add 300 μL APS, mix well, then add 30 μL TEMED, mix again, and quickly cast the gel. Insert an appropriate comb immediately without trapping air bubbles. Let the gel polymerize for at least 30 min.

3. After polymerization, place the gel into a vertical gel chamber, and fix it with metal clamps or clamps provided with the gel system. Remove the comb and wash the wells several times to remove residual urea (*see* **Note 8**).

4. Pre-run the gel for at least 15 min at 23 W (with 1× TBE as running buffer) with a metal plate attached to the front for equal heat distribution if possible.

5. Sample preparation: Add formamide loading buffer 1:1 to the RNA samples (1–20 μg total RNA in 5 μL DMPC-H_2O) as well as the DIG-labeled DNA ladder (2 μL, DIG VIII). Incubate for 2 min at 90 °C and place on ice. Briefly spin down before loading.

6. After the pre-run, remove the metal plate and wash the wells again. Load the samples and the DIG-labeled DNA ladder.

7. Attach the metal plate again and run the gel at 23 W for 1–2.5 h (depending on RNA sizes).

8. Prior to electroblotting, equilibrate the gel in 1× TBE blotting buffer for 5 min.

3.3 Membrane Transfer of Total RNA

The steps described in this section are similar for glyoxal agarose, as well as denaturing polyacrylamide Northern blotting.

1. Soak blotting paper and nylon membrane (according to the size of the gel) in 1× TBE blotting buffer for 5 min.

2. Assemble the transfer sandwich (as shown in Fig. 1b), starting with blotting paper (soaked in 1× TBE) on the anode metal plate. Cover the blotting paper with the nylon membrane and then place the gel on top of the membrane. To finish the transfer sandwich, use a second piece of soaked blotting paper (*see* **Note 9**).

3. Remove potentially trapped air bubbles, assemble the semidry electrophoretic transfer cell, and run the blot for 1 h at 15 V (limit to 3 mA/cm²).

4. After blotting, disassemble the transfer sandwich. Gently remove the gel and mark the orientation of the membrane by cutting one corner.

5. Transfer the membrane to a piece of Saran foil and cover it.

6. Cross-link the nucleic acids to the membrane with 120 mJ/cm² at 254 nm.

7. For glyoxal agarose Northern blots it is essential to remove the remaining glyoxal by incubation of the cross-linked membrane in 50 mM Tris–HCl pH 8.0 at 45 °C for 10 min before continuing with probe hybridization (*see* **Note 10**). Skip this step in denaturing polyacrylamide gel electrophoresis.

3.4 Northern Probe Design

Probe design is the first and maybe the most important step when planning a Northern blot experiment, in particular when circRNAs are detected. In general, different kind of probes can be used for Northern blot analysis, such as dsDNA probes, RNA probes, or oligonucleotide probes. However, since RNA antisense probes form stronger hybrids with the RNA target than DNA or oligonucleotides do, we will focus here only on the so-called riboprobes. RNA probes can be easily generated through transcription, either by runoff transcription or by using PCR-generated templates containing an RNA polymerase promoter sequence such as T7 or SP6.

Several things have to be considered when designing a probe for circRNAs:

1. Size: The size of the probe is critical for hybridization efficiency and background. For a low signal-to-noise ratio the minimum size should be 100 nt and usually not longer than 500 nt, since with longer probes the background signal may increase (*see* **Note 11**).

2. Sequence: In principle, the general rules for designing an antisense probe apply also to circRNA-specific probes. This implies for instance that the selected probe sequence should be

analyzed in terms of mispriming. In addition, the GC content should be between 40 and 60% to reach the optimal hybridization temperature of 68 °C for an RNA-RNA hybrid in formamide-based hybridization buffers.

For specifically detecting a circRNA by Northern blot, there are two options for probe design: using either a circ-junction specific probe or an exonic probe directed against a region within the circRNA (*see* Fig. 2a). The latter probe allows the simultaneous detection of a linear transcript (*see* Fig. 2b). When using exonic probes, further characterization is required to prove the circular configuration of the molecule analyzed (e.g., by RNase R and RNase H, *see* Subheadings 3.7 and 3.8).

3. Primer design for DIG-labeled riboprobes: Design primers to be used for riboprobe generation by following general guidelines for PCR primer design (*see* **Note 2**), attaching the T7 promoter sequence (5′-TAATACGACTCACTATAGGG-3′) or the SP6 promoter sequence (5′-ATTTAGGTGACACTATAG-3′) to the 5′-end of the reverse primer.

4. Antisense DNA oligonucleotides for RNase H cleavage: Oligonucleotides for RNase H assays can be designed like

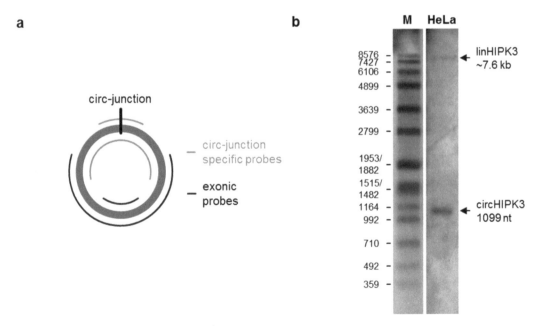

Fig. 2 Detection of circHIPK3 by glyoxal agarose Northern blot. (**a**) Schematic representation of possible positions for probes detecting circRNAs. These probes can be either circ-junction specific (covering the circ-junction sequence, light grey) or exonic (covering an internal sequence, black). Depending on the method used (DIG-labeled riboprobes or ^{32}P-labeled oligonucleotides), the size of the probe can vary. (**b**) Glyoxal agarose Northern blot detection of circHIPK3 (1099 nt) in HeLa total RNA (20 μg) with a DIG-labeled exonic riboprobe (covering the whole exon). In comparison to denaturing polyacrylamide gel electrophoresis (*see* Fig. 3), it is possible to additionally detect the linear isoform of HIPK3 (linHIPK3 ~7.6 kb) with this gel system. M, DIG-labeled DNA molecular weight marker VII

standard reverse primers (antisense to the target sequence, 18–22 nt) targeting either internal sequences or, if possible, the circ-junction of a target circRNA. Usually it is necessary to test a set of oligonucleotides for RNase H cleavage activity (*see* **Note 12**). Oligonucleotide-directed cleavage of a circRNA will result in a linearized product, which characteristically changes its running behavior in polyacrylamide gels (*see* Fig. 3 and **Note 13**). To conclusively confirm the circularity of a putative circRNA, it is recommended to combine two oligonucleotides targeting different sequences within the circRNA in one reaction. This will result in two circRNA-specific cleavage products that can be identified by size. It is essential to design the riboprobe such that it can detect all expected cleavage products by Northern blotting (*see* Figs. 2a and 3). Therefore it may be necessary to use a riboprobe covering the whole exon.

3.5 Detection of Specific circRNAs by DIG-labeled Probes

The steps described in this section are similar for both glyoxal agarose and denaturing polyacrylamide Northern blotting.

1. For glyoxal agarose Northern blotting, the additional step of glyoxal removal is essential (*see* Subheading 3.3, **step 7**).

2. For preparation of a DIG-labeled riboprobe, first reverse-transcribe RNA (according to the manufacturer's instructions) and subsequently perform a PCR reaction, using primers designed as described in Subheading 3.4.

3. After purification, the PCR product (with T7/SP6 promoter introduced) can be used as a template for DIG labeling by in vitro transcription (DIG RNA labeling mix, according to the manufacturer's instructions).

4. Digest the DNA template by adding DNase to the reaction (incubate for 30 min at 37 °C). Proceed with the purification of the transcribed riboprobe on RNA spin columns (as indicated in the manual, Roche).

5. Measure the concentration, check the size and quality by gel electrophoresis or with a Bioanalyzer, and store the riboprobe at −80 °C.

6. Pre-hybridization: Place the membrane in a hybridization tube, add 5–10 mL NorthernMax hybridization buffer (Roche), and incubate at 68 °C in a hybridization oven with constant rotation.

7. Hybridization: Denature the DIG-labeled riboprobe for 2 min at 95 °C and add the denatured probe to the hybridization buffer used for pre-hybridization (final concentration 25 ng/mL). Hybridize the probe overnight at 68 °C with constant rotation.

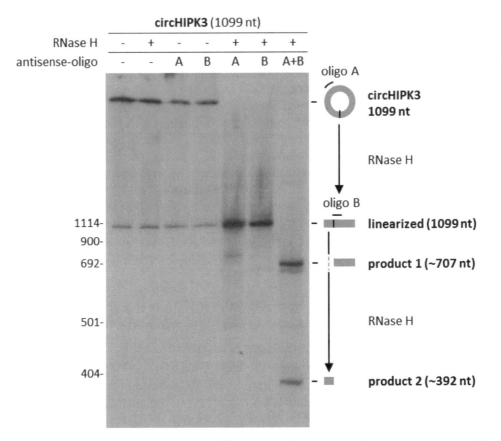

Fig. 3 Analysis of circular conformation of circHIPK3 by RNase H cleavage and Northern blot analysis. RNase H cleavage was performed with HeLa total RNA (as described in Subheading 3.4, **step 4**, and Subheading 3.8), using either a single antisense oligonucleotide (A or B) or a combination thereof (A + B). A schematic experimental outline is shown on the right side, including expected fragment sizes after RNase H cleavage reactions (sizes are approximate because the precise RNase H cleavage sites within the target region cannot be predicted). Additional controls were obtained in the absence of RNase H or oligonucleotide as indicated. RNA was analyzed on a 6% denaturing polyacrylamide gel and Northern blotting using a DIG-labeled exonic riboprobe for circHIPK3 (covering the whole exon, same as in Fig. 2b). The mobilities of circular and RNase H-linearized species, as well as the cleavage fragments (products 1 and 2), are indicated. Note that in this gel system no endogenous linear isoforms are detected, since they do not enter the gel. DIG-labeled DNA molecular weight marker VIII was used as size marker (modified from ref. [8] with permission from Elsevier)

8. Washing: Remove the hybridization buffer (containing the riboprobe) and add 25 mL of 2× SSC (supplemented with 0.1% SDS) washing buffer and rotate for 1 min.

9. Discard the buffer and wash again twice with 2× SSC (supplemented with 0.1% SDS) at 68 °C for 15 min.

10. Repeat the last steps by washing twice with 0.5× SSC (supplemented with 0.1% SDS).

11. Discard the SSC washing buffer and shortly equilibrate the membrane with DIG-washing buffer.

12. Blocking: Transfer the membrane to a tray into 2% DIG-blocking solution and incubate for 1 h shaking at room temperature.

13. Antibody binding: Add the anti-DIG-Fab fragment (coupled to alkaline phosphatase) to a final dilution of 1:10,000 to the DIG-blocking solution and continue the incubation at room temperature for 1 h while shaking.

14. Washing: Remove unbound antibody by washing the membrane in DIG-washing buffer, three times for 10 min, shaking (*see* **Note 14**).

15. Detection: Equilibrate the membrane in DIG-detection buffer for 2 min and transfer it to a plastic bag or Saran foil. Prepare 1 mL 0.5% CPD-star substrate solution (Roche) in DIG-detection buffer and add it to the plastic bag containing the membrane. Incubate for 5 min in the dark (*see* **Note 15**).

16. Remove excess of liquid without touching the membrane surface and seal plastic bag or Saran foil with adhesive tape.

17. For detection of the luminescence signals, place the membrane into a photo cassette and cover it with an X-ray film (in the dark, cut one corner to mark the orientation of the film). Expose for different time points (starting with 10 min).

18. Develop the exposed X-ray films with a processing machine.

3.6 Detection of Specific circRNAs by Radiolabeled Oligonucleotides

A good example of the usage of different types of short oligonucleotide probes to detect and characterize circRNAs is provided in ref. [14].

1. Due to lack of a marker in the detection procedure using radiolabeled oligonucleotides a standard marker should be used and ethidium bromide stained. To do so, an extra lane on one side of the gel should be used for markers, leaving sufficient space to the actual samples so that it can be cut off prior to blotting and stained by ethidium bromide (*see* **Note 16**).

2. Set up a 50 µL T4 polynucleotide kinase reaction according to the manufacturer's instructions, containing 25 pmol of the DNA oligonucleotide, followed by incubation for 1 h at 37 °C (*see* **Note 17**).

3. To get rid of free ^{32}P-ATP, perform gel filtration using mini Quick Spin Oligo Columns. Prepare columns by opening both ends and centrifuging for 1 min at $1000 \times g$ at room temperature. Place in new tube and load labeling reaction on column material (*see* **Note 18**). Spin for 4 min at $1000 \times g$ to elute the labeled oligonucleotides from the column. The volume of the sample will slightly increase to about 60–75 µL. The eluate can be directly used in Northern blot detection.

4. Use cross-linked membrane from Subheading 3.3, **steps 6** and 7, and place it into a pre-warmed hybridization tube filled with 5–10 mL of ULTRAhyb Ultrasensitive Hybridization Buffer. Pre-hybridization is performed for 1–2 h at 42 °C.

5. Radiolabeled oligonucleotide probe from steps 2 and 3 above is added to the hybridization buffer. Typically 1/5–1/10 of the reaction is used, containing 2.5–5 pmol of DNA oligonucleotide.

6. Hybridization is performed overnight at 42 °C (*see* **Note 19**).

7. Transfer the membrane to a tray and wash twice with 2× SSC (supplemented with 0.1% SDS) washing buffer for 10 min at room temperature.

8. Wash twice with 0.1× SSC (supplemented with 0.1% SDS) washing buffer for 10 min at room temperature (*see* **Note 20**).

9. For autoradiography, wrap membrane into Saran foil or plastic bag and expose either to an X-ray film at −80 °C, using an intensifier screen or to a phosphor imaging screen at room temperature.

10. Adjust stained marker lane to membrane edges on an overexposed autoradiogram.

3.7 Validation of circRNAs by RNase R Treatment

1. Prepare a reaction mix (typically 20–50 μL, with 1× RNase R buffer) containing the desired amount of total RNA to be analyzed (1–20 μg) and add 2.5 U of RNase R per μg RNA.

2. Incubate the reaction for 25 min at 37 °C.

3. Add DMPC-H_2O to the reaction to a total volume of 200 μL and proceed with standard phenol-chloroform extraction, followed by ethanol precipitation of the RNA.

4. Dissolve the RNA pellet in 5–10 μL DMPC-H_2O (depending on the downstream application).

5. Proceed with the steps described in Subheading 3.1 or 3.2 for Northern blot analysis (*see* **Note 21**).

3.8 Analysis of circRNAs by RNase H Cleavage

1. Prepare a reaction mix (typically 20–50 μL, with 1× RNase H buffer) containing the desired amount of total RNA to be analyzed (10 μg) as well as 2 μg antisense oligonucleotide (or a combination of two different oligonucleotides, *see* Subheading 3.4, point 4, and Fig. 3).

2. Incubate the reaction for 20 min at 37 °C (RNA-DNA hybrid formation, *see* **Note 22**).

3. Add 1 U of RNase H per μg RNA and continue the incubation for additional 40 min.

4. Add DMPC-H_2O to the reaction to a total volume of 200 μL and proceed with standard phenol-chloroform extraction, followed by ethanol precipitation of the RNA.

5. Dissolve the RNA pellet in 5 μL DMPC-H$_2$O.

6. Proceed with the steps described in Subheading 3.2 for Northern blot analysis by denaturing polyacrylamide gel electrophoresis. *See* ref. [15] for a detailed description on RNase H cleavage as an experimental tool.

4   Notes

1. DIG-blocking solution can be prepared as a 10% (w/v) blocking reagent stock solution (autoclave, store at 4 °C).

2. Design of oligonucleotide probes is comparable to PCR primer design. Mispriming/hybridization and extensive internal secondary structures should be avoided. Browser-based software employing mispriming libraries for several organisms is freely available to help with primer/probe design, e.g., Primer3 (http://primer3.ut.ee) [16].

3. This buffer system can be used without recirculation, which is an advantage in comparison to commonly used phosphate buffers that tend to form a pH gradient without recirculation.

4. Other dimensions can be used but gel thickness should not exceed 0.5 cm for efficient membrane transfer.

5. An advantage of this system over classical denaturing agarose gels with formaldehyde is that glyoxal is less toxic than formaldehyde.

6. This image can later be used for comparison with the DIG-labeled DNA size marker after blotting and anti-DIG detection.

7. Different gel systems may be used, ranging from minigel systems (7.5 × 10 cm) to large gels (e.g., 20 × 20 cm). The spacer thickness should not exceed 0.75 mm.

8. The wells should be washed thoroughly and cleared of residual polyacrylamide pieces. These can be removed with a thin-gauged needle or piece of X-ray film cut to fit.

9. Transferring thin 6% polyacrylamide gels can be difficult. Try not to apply too much sheer forces to the gel. This will result in odd shape of lanes/bands. Use excess of 1× TBE buffer in every step and transfer gel with the help of an X-ray film or a transparency foil. First transfer the gel to the foil (let it slide onto the foil just by gravity), and then from the foil to the membrane. Bending the foil helps releasing the gel.

10. This step reverses the denaturing effect of glyoxal reacting with guanosine residues in the RNA.

11. Smaller riboprobes can be used as well (30–100 nt); however one has to consider the way of labeling the probe (e.g., sufficient

number of uridine nucleotides necessary for labeling by DIG-UTP) and that the background level can increase significantly. Longer probes (depending on the circRNA target size) may be used for RNase H assays.

12. This step may be necessary since different target regions often vary in accessibility for antisense oligonucleotides. Besides that it should be noted that it is not always possible to use oligonucleotides against the circ-junction due to possible sequence similarities with other unrelated sequences (BLAST analysis is highly recommended when designing antisense oligonucleotides).

13. Since circRNAs show aberrant running behavior in polyacrylamide gels (which is not the case for agarose gels, *see* Fig. 2b), a linearized circRNA molecule can be identified by the expected size, while circular molecules usually run at size ranges higher than expected from linear markers.

14. Changing trays after DIG antibody incubation can reduce background.

15. For optimization of the signal-to-noise ratio the substrate concentration can be lowered (0.2–0.1%) if a solid specific signal is obtained.

16. Cutting the membrane to exactly fit the gel height before blotting helps to adjust the markers after autoradiography.

17. T4 polynucleotide kinase requires a minimum final concentration of 1 pmol/μL of ATP in the reaction mix to work efficiently.

18. It is crucial to load the sample directly on the column material without touching the side of the tube; otherwise free ^{32}P-ATP will remain in your sample instead of being retained on the column.

19. Depending on the specificity of the probe and background obtained, the hybridization temperatures can be altered. Consider that the formamide in the hybridization buffer lowers the annealing temperature of the probes, so that the calculated melting temperatures of the oligonucleotides do not apply. Increase temperature if the background is too high, and lower temperature if the specific signal is too low. For more specificity, perform pre-hybridization at higher temperature (maximum 65 °C), add the probe, and set the hybridization oven to a lower temperature (30–42 °C), so it slowly cools down during overnight incubation.

20. Decreasing the salt concentration gradually will remove unspecifically bound probes.

21. For this kind of experiment a "linear control" should be considered (detection of a linear mRNA isoform) to confirm that the RNase R treatment was successful.

22. Other temperatures may be tested for oligonucleotide hybridization; however, we found that 37 °C works best in most cases.

Acknowledgments

This work was supported by the LOEWE program "Medical RNomics" (State of Hessen; to A.B. and O.R.) and by grants from the Deutsche Forschungsgemeinschaft (to A.B.). We would like to thank Roland Hartmann for advice on Northern detection by oligonucleotide probes, and Nikolaus Rajewsky, Jørgen Kjems, and members of our laboratory for discussions.

References

1. Lasda E, Parker R (2014) Circular RNAs: diversity of form and function. RNA 20:1829–1842

2. Chen LL (2016) The biogenesis and emerging roles of circular RNAs. Nat Rev Mol Cell Biol 17:205–211

3. Sanger HL, Klotz G, Riesner D, Gross HJ, Kleinschmidt AK (1976) Viroids are single-stranded covalently closed circular RNA molecules existing as highly base-paired rod-like structures. Proc Natl Acad Sci U S A 73:3852–3856

4. Salzman J, Gawad C, Wang PL, Lacayo N, Brown PO (2012) Circular RNAs are the predominant transcript isoform from hundreds of human genes in diverse cell types. PLoS One 7:e30733

5. Jeck WR, Sorrentino JA, Wang K, Slevin MK, Burd CE, Liu J, Marzluff WF, Sharpless NE (2013) Circular RNAs are abundant, conserved, and associated with ALU repeats. RNA 19:141–157

6. Memczak S, Jens M, Elefsinioti A, Torti F, Krueger J, Rybak A, Maier L, Mackowiak SD, Gregersen LH, Munschauer M, Loewer A, Ziebold U, Landthaler M, Kocks C, le Noble F, Rajewsky N (2013) Circular RNAs are a large class of animal RNAs with regulatory potency. Nature 495:333–338

7. Hansen TB, Jensen TI, Clausen BH, Bramsen JB, Finsen B, Damgaard CK, Kjems J (2013) Natural RNA circles function as efficient microRNA sponges. Nature 495:384–388

8. Starke S, Jost I, Rossbach O, Schneider T, Schreiner S, Hung LH, Bindereif A (2015) Exon circularization requires canonical splice signals. Cell Rep 10:103–111

9. Tabak HF, Van der Horst G, Smit J, Winter AJ, Mul Y, Groot Koerkamp MJ (1988) Discrimination between RNA circles, interlocked RNA circles and lariats using two-dimensional polyacrylamide gel electrophoresis. Nucleic Acids Res 16:6597–6605

10. McMaster GK, Carmichael GG (1977) Analysis of single- and double-stranded nucleic acids on polyacrylamide and agarose gels by using glyoxal and acridine orange. Proc Natl Acad Sci U S A 74:4835–4838

11. Thomas PS (1980) Hybridization of denatured RNA and small DNA fragments transferred to nitrocellulose. Proc Natl Acad Sci U S A 77:5201–5205

12. Burnett WV (1997) Northern blotting of RNA denatured in glyoxal without buffer recirculation. Biotechniques 22:668–671

13. Behm-Ansmant I, Helm M, Motorin Y (2011) Use of specific chemical reagents for detection of modified nucleotides in RNA. J Nucleic Acids 2011:408053

14. Kramer MC, Liang D, Tatomer DC, Gold B, March ZM, Cherry S, Wilusz JE (2015) Combinatorial control of Drosophila circular RNA expression by intronic repeats, hnRNPs, and SR proteins. Genes Dev 29:2168–2182

15. Günzl A, Palfi Z, Bindereif A (2002) Analysis of RNA-protein complexes by oligonucleotide-targeted RNase H digestion. Methods 26:162–169

16. Untergasser A, Cutcutache I, Koressaar T, Ye J, Faircloth BC, Remm M, Rozen SG (2012) Primer3 - new capabilities and interfaces. Nucleic Acids Res 40:e115

Chapter 11

Nonradioactive Northern Blot of circRNAs

Xiaolin Wang and Ge Shan

Abstract

Circular RNAs (circRNAs) are recognized as a special species of transcripts in metazoans with increasing studies, and northern blotting is a direct way to confirm the existence and to evaluate the size of individual circRNAs. Northern blotting probes can be radioactive isotope (^{32}P) labeled, which is not environment-friendly and sometimes inconvenient to use. Here, we describe a nonradioactive northern blot protocol with digoxigenin-labeled probe to detect circRNA.

Key words Nonradioactive, Northern blot, circRNA, Digoxigenin

1 Introduction

Covalently closed circular RNAs (circRNAs) were firstly discovered in plant viroids and later hepatitis delta virus in 1970s [1, 2]. Owning to the advance of high-throughput RNA sequencing and bioinformatics, circRNAs have been gradually recognized as a special class of RNAs in eukaryotic cells [3–7]. When studying circRNA, it is important to confirm experimentally the existence of individual circRNAs. Northern blotting is almost the most convincing approach to examine the existence, abundance, and size of circRNA.

A general northern blotting procedure [8] starts with denatured RNA samples separated by gel electrophoresis. Then the RNAs separated by size are transferred to nylon membrane through capillary or electrical means. Once transfer is finished, RNAs are immobilized through covalent linkage to the membrane by UV light or baking. The labeled probe against specific RNA sequences is then hybridized with the membrane. After washing the membrane, the hybrid signals are then detected with various methods depending on the way of probe labeling.

Classically probes of northern blotting were labeled with radioactive isotopes, mostly ^{32}P [4, 6]. Since radioactive materials are potentially harmful to health and environment, and relatively hard to handle or recycle [9], nonradioactive-labeled probes are

Christoph Dieterich and Argyris Papantonis (eds.), *Circular RNAs: Methods and Protocols*, Methods in Molecular Biology, vol. 1724, https://doi.org/10.1007/978-1-4939-7562-4_11, © Springer Science+Business Media, LLC 2018

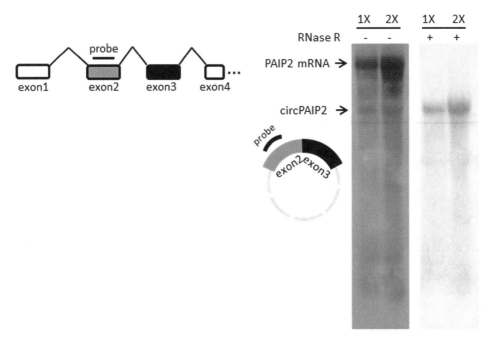

Fig. 1 Image of nonradioactive northern blot of circPAIP2. Sequence composition of PAIP2 mRNA and circRNA with position of the probe are indicated

thus good alternatives [10]. Here, we describe the nonradioactive northern blot for circRNAs with digoxigenin-labeled probe. One probe is designed to detect the circPAIP2 in this particular experiment (Fig. 1) [10]. RNase R is a RNA exonuclease that can degrade linear RNA and keep the circRNA intact, and it is now commonly used to verify the RNA as covalently closed molecule.

2   Materials

Prepare all solutions with RNase-free water, which is purified deionized water pretreated by 0.1% DEPC with autoclave. All compounds used are analytical grade. Filter all solutions through a 0.22 μm Corning filter before use. Prepare and store all reagents at room temperature (unless otherwise specified). Diligently follow all waste disposal requirements when disposing waste materials.

1. 10× MOPS buffer: 4 mol/L 3-(4-Morpholino) propanesulfonic acid (MOPS), 1 mol/L NaOAc, 100 mol/L EDTA, pH 7.0. Weigh 92.4 g MOPS, 13.6 g NaOAc, 7.6 g EDTA, and transfer them to the beaker (*see* **Note 1**). Add RNase-free water to a volume of 900 mL. Mix and adjust pH with NaOH (Add around 8 g) (*see* **Note 2**). Make up to 1 L, filter, and autoclave. Store the buffer in brown bottle to avoid decomposing at 4 °C (*see* **Note 3**).

2. Agarose.

3. Gelred (nucleic acid dye).

4. 37% formaldehyde (*see* **Note 4**).

5. 2× loading buffer.

6. 10× TBE buffer: 0.9 mol/L Tris-borieacid, 0.02 mol/L EDTA, pH 8.3. Weigh 108 g Tris base, 9.2 g EDTA, 55.2 g borieacid, and transfer them to the beaker. Add RNase-free water to a volume of 900 mL. Mix and adjust pH with HCl. Make up to 1 L, filter and autoclave. Store the buffer at room temperature (*see* **Note 5**).

7. Nylon membranes.

8. Labeling mix.

9. Transcription buffer.

10. T7 RNA polymerase.

11. DNase I enzyme.
    8–11 (*see* **Note 6**) were included in Roche DIG RNA Labeling Kit.

12. 20× SSC buffer: 3 mol/L NaCl, 0.3 mol/L sodium citrate, pH 7.0. Weigh 175.3 g NaCl, 88.2 g sodium citrate, and transfer them to the beaker. Add RNase-free water to a volume of 900 mL. Mix and adjust pH with NaOH. Make up to 1 L and filter. Store the buffer at room temperature.

13. 10% SDS: Weigh 10 g SDS and transfer them to the beaker. Add RNase-free water to a volume of 100 mL. Mix, filter, and store the buffer at room temperature (*see* **Note 7**).

14. Washing buffer I: 2× SSC, 0.1%SDS.

15. Washing buffer II: 0.5× SSC, 0.1%SDS.

16. Maleic acid buffer: 0.1 mol/L Maleic acid, 0.15 mol/L NaCl, pH 7.5. Weigh 11.6 g maleic acid, 8.8 g NaCl, and transfer them to the beaker. Add RNase-free water to a volume of 900 mL. Mix and adjust pH with NaOH. Make up to 1 L and filter. Store the buffer at room temperature.

17. Washing buffer: 100 mL Maleic acid buffer add 300 μL Tween 20 (*see* **Note 8**).

18. Detection buffer: 0.1 mol/L Tris–HCl, 0.1 mol/L NaCl, pH 9.5. Weigh 12.1 g Tris base, 5.8 g NaCl, and transfer them to the beaker. Add RNase-free water to a volume of 900 mL. Mix and adjust pH with NaOH. Make up to 1 L and filter. Store the buffer at room temperature.

19. Anti-digoxigenin-AP, Fab fragments (*see* **Note 9**).

20. CDP-Star (the Chemiluminescent Substrate), ready-to-use.

21. DIG Easy Hyb Granules (*see* **Note 10**).

22. Blocking solution.
    19–22 were included in DIG Northern Starter Kit.

3 Methods

Carry out all the procedures at room temperature unless specified.

3.1 1% Formaldehyde Agarose Gel

The concentration of the gel for the length of RNA <1000 nt is 1.5% and ≥1000 nt is 1%.

1. Prepare an 1% agarose gel (50 mL) by mixing 0.5 g agarose with 43.5 mL RNase-free water.

2. Microwave the mixture into solution and cool to 55 °C in water bath.

3. Add 5 μL Gelred (10,000×), 5 mL 10× MOPS, and 1.5 mL 37% formaldehyde for the final concentrations of 1×, 1×, and 1%, respectively (*see* **Note 11**).

4. Mix and pour the gel in the hood to avoid toxic formaldehyde fume.

5. Let the gel sit for at least half an hour in hood before use.

3.2 Electrophoresis and Membrane Transfer of RNA

1. Mix RNA samples (10–30 μg total RNA per lane) and 2× loading buffer in tubes.

2. Heat samples at 80 °C for 10 min to denature RNA (*see* **Note 12**), and then place in ice water immediately.

3. Spin samples briefly and load on the gel (*see* **Note 13**).

4. Run the gel at 150 V for 1 h with recirculating buffer (1× MOPS) and take photos (*see* **Note 14**).

5. Soak the gel in a large volume of RNase-free water with gentle shaking to remove the formaldehyde and carefully pre-wet the membrane in RNase-free water for 5 min.

6. Transfer the RNA from the gel to a membrane with wet transfer using 0.5× TBE buffer at 200 mA overnight (*see* **Note 15**).

3.3 Nonradioactive Probe Preparation

1. Design the probe. For circRNA, two kinds of probes can be selected. One is against the continuous exon region. Another kind is against the exon-exon junction of circRNA. Length of the probe is generally 100–200 nt.

2. Prepare the template. The T7 promoter sequences (*see* **Note 16**) are added to PCR primers, and thus are incorporated into the PCR products.

3. Synthesize the digoxigenin-labeled (DIG-labeled) RNA probe by mixing together the following components (Roche DIG RNA Labeling Kit).

   (a) 1 μg DNA template (*see* **Note 17**).

   (b) 4 μL Labeling mix.

(c) 4 μL Transcription buffer.

(d) 2 μL T7 RNA polymerase.

(e) Add RNase-free water to 20 μL.

4. Incubate the mixture at 37 °C for 4 h instead of overnight, then with 1 μL DNase I incubation for 15 min to remove the DNA template.

5. Purify the probe with trizol extraction (Life Technologies) and confirm with RNA gel.

3.4 Hybridization

1. Crosslink RNA to nylon membrane which prefers wet membrane with 2× SSC buffer using UV and dry at 80 °C for 1 h in a hybridization oven.

2. Pre-hybridize with pre-heated DIG Easy Hyb buffer for 2 h with gentle agitation in an appropriate container (*see* **Note 18**).

3. Denature 100 pmol DIG-labeled RNA probe by boiling for 10 min and rapidly cooling in ice water.

4. Mix the denatured DIG-labeled RNA probe with pre-heated DIG Easy Hyb buffer (avoid foaming).

5. Hybridize at 45–68 °C overnight with gentle agitation in a hybridization oven.

3.5 Detection

All the following procedures are according to the protocol of DIG Northern Starter Kit with some modifications.

1. Wash the membrane for 5 min in ample Washing buffer I at 15–25 °C under constant agitation, twice.

2. Wash the membrane for 15 min in ample Washing buffer II at 45–68 °C under constant agitation, twice. These four washes are stringency washes.

3. Rinse the membrane briefly for 5 min in Washing buffer.

4. Incubate the membrane with 10 mL Blocking solution for 1 h.

5. Incubate the membrane with 10 mL Antibody solution (1 μL Anti-digoxigenin-AP antibody diluted in 10 mL Blocking solution) for 1 h.

6. Wash the membrane for 15 min in Washing buffer, twice and equilibrate the membrane in 20 mL Detection buffer for 5 min.

7. Cover the membrane with ample CSPD ready-to-use immediately, and incubate for 10–30 min at 37 °C to enhance the luminescent reaction (*see* **Note 19**).

8. Expose the membrane and take images with an appropriate imager (e.g., ImageQuant LAS4000 Biomolecular Imager, expose for 5–20 min for detection).

4 Notes

1. Adding some water into the beaker first and with magnetic stir bar working help to dissolve the MOPS.

2. When adjusting pH, high concentrated HCl or NaOH can be used firstly to shorten the gap from the starting pH to the required pH. Then the HCl or NaOH of lower ionic strengths could be used until up to the required pH.

3. MOPS buffer is susceptible to bacterial contamination and light decomposition. It is not suitable for experimental use when the color is light yellow.

4. When dealing with formaldehyde, all handling must be in fume hood.

5. 10× TBE is very easy to precipitate, even when it is stored at the room temperature. Stir with magnetic bar in a 37 °C water bath to fully dissolve the solution before use.

6. All the components must be stored at −20 °C and avoid alternate freezing.

7. Do not place 10% SDS on ice, because of its rapid and easy precipitation at low temperature.

8. Tween 20 is very viscous and susceptible to sticking on the pipette; using pipettes with tips cut to aliquot Tween 20 is essential.

9. Centrifuge before use.

10. Add 64 mL RNase-free water into DIG Easy Hyb granule immediately. DIG Easy Hyb solution is stable at the room temperature for 1 month.

11. Gelred, 10× MOPS, and 37% formaldehyde can mix together and pre-warm in a 55 °C water bath. And then add the mixture along the wall of the glass beaker to avoid solidification and foaming.

12. Denature the samples at 100 °C for 5 min, which can disrupt the RNA secondary structure.

13. The suggested volume is no more than 60 μL, and the maximum amount of total RNA is 50 μg per lane.

14. Run the gel briefly for 10–15 min; taking photos to visualize ribosomal RNA bands helps to show equal loading of total RNAs.

15. Use fresh diluted 0.5× TBE transfer buffer. Wet transfer needs to be carried out in ice water bath.

16. When designing the primer, make sure the T7 promoter sequence TAATACGACTCACTATAGGG was added, so that this sequence is in 5′ of the antisense strand to the interested

RNA. The first 17 nt is the core region of T7 promoter. The three Gs followed can enhance the transcriptional efficiency.

17. The templates need to be purified with Gel cycle and dry in air for longer time (~20 min) to remove moisture completely, and this can enhance the transcriptional efficiency.

18. UVP molecular hybrid tube is recommended for pre-hybridization. And bubbles between the membrane and the wall of hybrid tube need to be avoided to decrease background.

19. Appropriate increase of the incubation time in "CSPD ready-to-use" can sometimes get clearer image.

Acknowledgments

This work was supported by the National Basic Research Program of China (2015CB943000), National Natural Science Foundation of China (31471225), and the Fundamental Research Funds for the Central Universities (WK2070000034).

References

1. Sanger HL, Klotz G, Riesner D et al (1976) Viroids are single-stranded covalently closed circular RNA molecules existing as highly base-paired rod-like structures. Proc Natl Acad Sci U S A 73(11):3852–3856

2. Kos A, Dijkema R, Arnberg AC, van der Meide PH, Schellekens H (1986) The hepatitis delta (delta) virus possesses a circular RNA. Nature 323:558–560

3. Dixon RJ, Eperon IC, Hall L, Samani NJ (2005) A genome-wide survey demonstrates widespread non-linear mRNA in expressed sequences from multiple species. Nucleic Acids Res 33:5904–5913

4. Hansen TB et al (2013) Natural RNA circles function as efficient microRNA sponges. Nature 495:384–388

5. Jeck WR et al (2013) Circular RNAs are abundant, conserved, and associated with ALU repeats. RNA 19:141–157

6. Memczak S et al (2013) Circular RNAs are a large class of animal RNAs with regulatory potency. Nature 495:333–338

7. Salzman J, Chen RE, Olsen MN, Wang PL, Brown PO (2013) Cell-type specific features of circular RNA expression. PLoS Genet 9: e1003777

8. Trayhurn P (1996) Northern blotting. Pro Nutr Soc 55:583–589

9. Streit S, Michalski CW, Erkan M, Kleeff J, Friess H (2009) Northern blot analysis for detection and quantification of RNA in pancreatic cancer cells and tissues. Nat Protoc 4(1):37–43

10. Li Z et al (2015) Exon-intron circular RNAs regulate transcription in the nucleus. Nat Struct Mol Biol 22:2959

Chapter 12

Characterization of Circular RNA Concatemers

Thomas B. Hansen

Abstract

Circular RNAs (circRNAs) constitute a novel subset in the fascinating world of noncoding RNA, and they are found in practically all eukaryotes. Most of them exhibit low expression levels but some are extremely abundant. Typically, circRNAs are studied by RT-PCR-based assays, but for certain types of analyses this technique is not suitable. Circular RNA with repetitive exons (circular concatemers) has been observed by us and others when transiently expressing circRNAs in cells, however techniques and assays to study these species have not been established. Here, this chapter outlines three biochemical assays (RNase R-, RNase H-, and alkaline-treatment) that combined with northern blotting are useful to study circRNAs in general and circular RNA concatemers in particular.

Key words Circular RNA, RNA concatemers, RNAse R, RNAse H, Alkaline treatment, Northern blotting

---

1 Introduction

One of the most recent discoveries in the world of noncoding RNA is the existence of circular RNA (circRNA, reviewed in [1]). These RNA species are produced by a nonlinear back-splicing event connecting a downstream splice donor with an upstream splice acceptor. CircRNAs have been found in all eukaryotes investigated and it is already well established that several thousand different circRNAs exist in humans. For the vast majority, the functional relevance is unclear, however a small subset of circRNAs has been shown to act as decoys for miRNAs [2–4] or to bind and regulate protein function [5, 6].

Backsplicing has been shown to be stimulated by flanking inverted repeats [2, 7–9]. This is often facilitated by inverted *Alu* elements in humans [10], but based on circRNA-producing vectors, sequences of any origin seem to have the ability to stimulate circularization as long as they are inverted [2, 9]. The current model on circRNA biogenesis proposes that the inverted repeats engage in base-pairing, thereby positioning the two splicesites in

Christoph Dieterich and Argyris Papantonis (eds.), *Circular RNAs: Methods and Protocols*, Methods in Molecular Biology, vol. 1724, https://doi.org/10.1007/978-1-4939-7562-4_12, © Springer Science+Business Media, LLC 2018

close proximity (Fig. 1a). One design we have constructed in the lab, is the encapsulation of exon 2 from beta-globin (HBB) in-between inverted elements (as depicted in Fig. 1b). To our knowledge, this exon is not producing circRNA in its natural context, but when flanked with inverted repeats, the exon not only produces one distinct circRNA, but a ladder of circRNA-like products (circRNA concatemers; *see* Fig. 1b–d). Whether this ladder of circRNA species is biologically relevant or an artifact of vector-based overexpression is currently unknown, and this will not be discussed further in this chapter, however techniques to accurately characterize circRNA concatemers have not been established.

The detection and profiling of circRNA is typically done by next-generation sequencing (NGS) or by qRT-PCR [11–13]. In both cases the NGS read or the PCR amplicon used is spanning the back-splice junction (BSJ) to specifically demarcate circular RNA from overlapping linear mRNAs. While these techniques are powerful, sensitive and versatile, and suitable for most types of analyses, particular questions cannot be answered by these approaches. Basically, a reverse transcription (RT) step is required for both RNA sequencing and qRT-PCR. Reverse transcriptases are very prone to template switching [14] and in some unfortunate cases, this leads to false positive identification of circRNAs. Moreover, and importantly, reverse transcription on circRNA templates generates concatemeric cDNA by "rolling circle" amplification [15, 16], and this obscures whether the circRNA to begin with contained exon repeats or whether the repetitiveness was introduced by the RT enzyme. Instead, we here outline simple biochemical assays visualized by northern blotting to study the nature of these circRNAs and to show that they are indeed composed of exon repeats (circRNA concatemers). This involves three distinct experiments: (1) An RNase R digestion (Fig. 1b, Subheading 3.2) to validate the circular structure of the circRNA species. (2) An RNase H digestion (Fig. 1c, Subheading 3.3) to determine the composition of exons by collapsing the circRNAs into their comprising exon-units. And finally (3) An alkaline treatment (Fig. 1d, Subheading 3.4) to gently nick the circRNA into a corresponding linear RNA, thereby distinguishing between concatemers and intertwined circRNAs (topologically locked single exon circRNAs, *see* Fig. 1a).

2   Materials

2.1 circRNA Biochemistry

1. H_2O: Nuclease-free water or DEPC-treated water.
2. Temperature adjustable thermoblock.
3. Purified total RNA (1 g/L) (*see* **Note 1**).
4. RNase-free tubes and filter tips.

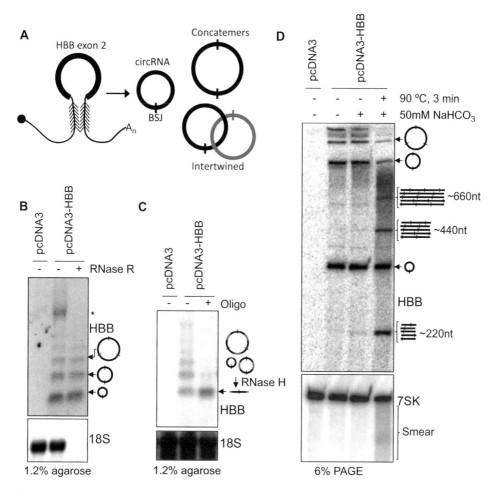

Fig. 1 Characterization of circRNA concatemers. (**a**) Schematic representation of circHBB biogenesis. Exon 2 (223 nt; chr11:5247807-5248029(-);hg19) from beta-globin is flanked by inverted repeats (*arrowheads*). Upon transcription, the inverted repeats position the splice sites in close proximity, thereby stimulating back-splicing and circular RNA production. To distinguish monomeric from concatameric circRNA, the backsplice junction (BSJ) is marked with a perpendicular line traversing the circle. Also, as a hypothetical scenario, two topologically joined ("Intertwined") circRNAs colored *black* and *gray*, respectively, are depicted. (**b** and **c**) 1.2% agarose northern with RNA derived from HEK293 cells transiently transfected with either an empty vector (pcDNA3) or the circHBB expression vector (pcDNA3-HBB) subjected to RNase R digest (**b**) or RNase H digest (**c**) as denoted. For (**b**) the RNase R resistant bands are marked to the *right* with the corresponding circRNA. For (**c**) the DNA antisense oligo target sequence is illustrated in *red*, and the RNAse H-mediated collapse of circRNA into one monomeric exon is marked with *arrow* to the *right*. *Upper panel* and *lower panel* are probed for HBB exon 2 and 18S, respectively. (**d**) Alkaline treatment of RNA derived from HEK293 cells transiently transfected with either an empty vector (pcDNA3) or the circHBB expression vector (pcDNA3-HBB). The RNA has been separated on a 6% PAGE and probed for HBB and 7SK as denoted. As in (**b** and **c**) the repetitive nature of the circRNAs is illustrated by BSJ-representing dashes. Upon alkaline treatment, random nicking of circRNAs produces linear RNA species with distinct length; ~220 nt, ~440 nt, or ~660 nt for mono-, di-, and tri-meric circRNA concatemers, respectively

5. RNase R (20 U/μL, Epicentre) with 10× Reaction Buffer: 0.2 M Tris–HCl (pH 8.0), 1 M KCl, and 1 mM $MgCl_2$.

6. Ribolock RNase Inhibitor (40 U/μL, Thermo Scientific).

7. RNase H (2 U/μL, Invitrogen) with 5× Reaction Buffer: 200 mM Tris (pH 7.5), 1 M KCl, 100 mM $MgCl_2$, 1 mM DTT.

8. DNA antisense oligo (10 μM), here we use: 5′-CAGCATCAGGAGTGGACAGA-3′.

9. Ribolock RNase Inhibitor (40 U/μL, Thermo Scientific).

10. 100 mM $NaHCO_3$ (pH 9).

2.2 Northern Blotting (Agarose and PAGE)

2.2.1 General

1. Power supplies.

2. Hot plate with magnetic stirrer.

3. Hybridization oven and tubes.

4. UV gel image system.

5. Phosphoimager screens and scanner.

6. Bench type Geiger–Müller counter with end-window detector.

2.2.2 Agarose Gel

1. Agarose.

2. 50× MOPS: 1 M MOPS, 0.25 M NaOAc, 50 mM EDTA, pH 7. Pass the buffer through a sterile filter and wrap in aluminum foil to avoid direct exposure to light. Keep at 4 °C.

3. 37% Formaldehyde.

4. Formamide Loading Buffer: 500 μL formamide, 150 μL 37% formaldehyde, 20 μL 50× MOPS, 16 μL 0.6 mg/mL ethidium Bromide, 165 μL H_2O, 0.025% bromophenol blue.

5. 20× SSC: 3 M NaCl, 0.3 M Na_3Citrate (pH 7).

6. Horizontal submerged gel-electrophoresis apparatus.

2.2.3 PAGE (Polyacrylamide Gel Electrophoresis)

1. SequaGel—UreaGel System (National Diagnostics).

2. N,N,N′,N′-Tetramethyl ethylenediamine (TEMED).

3. 10% Ammonium persulfate (APS). Keep at 4 °C.

4. 10× TBE: 890 mM Tris, 890 mM boric acid, 20 mM EDTA.

5. 96% ethanol.

6. 3 M NaOAc.

7. Glycogen (20 g/L). Keep at −20 °C.

8. Centrifuge at 4 °C.

9. Urea Loading Buffer: 8 M Urea, 20 mM EDTA, 0.025% bromophenol blue.

10. Ethidium bromide stain: 2 mg/mL ethidium bromide in 0.5× TBE.

Table 1
Northern blotting probes

Probe	Sequence (5′-3′)
HBB	AAAGGTGCCCTTGAGGTTGTCCAGGTGAGCCAGGCCATCACTAAAGGCAC CGAGCACTTT
18S	TTACCGCGGCTGCTGGCACCAGACTTGCCCTCCAATGGATCCTCGTTAAAG GATTTAAAGTGGACTCATTCCAATTACAG
7SK	TACTCGTATACCCTTGACCGAAGACCGGTCCTCCTCTATCGGGGATGGTC

11. Vertical gel-electrophoresis apparatus with plates, spacers, and comb.

12. Trans-Blot® Cell with Plate Electrodes with gel cassettes and foam pads (Bio-Rad), or other commercially available wet-transfer setup.

2.2.4 Transfer, Hybridization, and Exposure

1. N+ Hybond™ membranes (GE Healthcare).

2. Crosslinker (e.g., UVP CL-1000 crosslinker, 254 nm, shortwave).

3. T4 Polynucleotide Kinase (10 U/μL, Thermo scientific) with 10× Reaction buffer A: 500 mM Tris–HCl (pH 7.6), 100 mM $MgCl_2$, 50 mM DTT, 1 mM spermidine. Other commercially available T4 Polynucleotide Kinases can also be used.

4. DNA Probe (10 μM). The probes used here are listed in Table 1 (*see* **Note 2**).

5. [y-32P]ATP (10 mCi/mL, 3000 Ci/mmol).

6. G50 Columns (GE Healthcare).

7. Church Buffer: 0.5 M $NaPO_4$ (0.158 M NaH_2PO_4 + 0.342 M Na_2HPO_4, pH 7.5), 1 mM EDTA, 0.5% BSA, 7% SDS. To dissolve, heat to 65 °C while on magnetic stirrer.

8. Washing Solution #1: 2× SSC, 0.1% SDS.

9. Washing Solution #2: 0.2× SSC, 0.1% SDS.

10. Stripping Solution: 1 mM EDTA, 0.1% SDS.

3 Methods

3.1 General Considerations

It is imperative that all procedures are carried out using nuclease-free or DEPC-treated water. When working with RNA, always protect samples carefully by working on a clean bench with gloves and filter-tips. For long storage, keep RNA on −80 °C, and while handling RNA always keep on ice unless incubating (*see* **Note 1**).

Table 2
RNase R digest

	Pos. (μL)	Neg. (μL)
10× RNase R reaction buffer	1	1
Ribolock RNase inhibitor	0.5	0.5
H_2O	3	3.5
RNA (1 μg/ μL)	5	5

The three biochemical assays outlined below (Subheadings 3.2–3.4) are not very time consuming and could easily be completed in half a day. The subsequent northern blotting, however, has two overnight steps which makes it a rather sturdy technique, although the hands-on time is manageable. Therefore, we recommend collecting and combining as many samples as possible on the northern gel to increase the efficiency and output (*see* **Note 3**).

3.2   RNase R

The most common approach to validate the nonlinear topology of circRNAs is by using RNase R, a 3′ exonuclease [17, 18]. Here, circular RNAs are resistant and should therefore be unaffected by the treatment in contrast to the vast majority of linear RNAs (Fig. 1c, *see* **Note 4**).

1. For each RNA sample prepare the following in ice (Table 2) (*see* **Notes 5–7**).

2. Heat samples briefly to 95 °C for 30 s and cool instantly on ice (*see* **Note 8**).

3. Add 0.5 μL RNase R to the enzyme-positive reaction (*see* **Note 9**).

4. Incubate at 37 °C for 10 min.

5. After incubation, proceed directly to northern blotting by adding 20 μL Formamide Loading Buffer to the samples (*see* Subheading 3.6, **step 3**) (*see* **Note 10**).

3.3   RNase H Digest

Before RNase R became commercially available, RNase H digestion was a suitable technique to determine the circular topology of RNA, e.g., for circSry [19]. RNase H acts on RNA:DNA hybrids which in the laboratory can be harnessed by directing the RNase H enzyme to RNA of choice using a short antisense DNA oligo. Here, in the context of circRNA concatemers, we use RNase R digest to validate that the circRNA species seen by northern blotting in fact comprise only one exon unit. In case of exon concatemerization, RNase H will specifically cleave all exon repeats harboring a cognate complementary sequence to the DNA antisense oligo, thereby collapsing the series of concatemers into the size of the exon unit (Fig. 1c).

Table 3
The RNase H reaction

	Pos. (µL)	Neg. (µL)
5× RNase H reaction buffer	5	5
Ribolock RNase inhibitor	1	1
H_2O	32	33
DNA antisense oligo (10 µM)	1	0
RNA (1 µg/µL)	10	10

1. For each RNase H reaction, prepare the following on ice (Table 3) (*see* **Notes 5–7**).

2. Incubate reaction at 75 °C for 5 min, then 37 °C for 30 min to anneal the oligo to the RNA.

3. Add 1 µL RNase H to all tubes.

4. Incubate at 37 °C for 30 min.

5. After incubation, precipitate all samples (*see* Subheading 3.5).

3.4 Alkaline Hydrolysis

The following protocol is for random nicking of RNA using alkaline hydrolysis [20]. For circRNA, irrespective of where in the sequence the nicking occurs, the length of the resulting linear RNA will correspond to the length of the circRNA from which it derives. Therefore, nicking of circRNAs produces distinct linear species in contrast to the smear produced by nicking of linear RNA. This makes it possible to demarcate concatemers from intertwined circRNAs (*see* Fig. 1a), as the circRNA concatemers should also produce linear concatemers upon alkaline treatment (Fig. 1d). To distinguish between circular and linear RNA, the alkaline treatment must be separated on a high percent PAGE (here we use 6%), where circRNA migration is retarded [21]. The procedure is a very easy and cost-effective approach to study circular RNA. The hydrolysis is conducted by heating RNA in the presence of a mild alkaline solution. The limitation is that a rather high percentage gel is required for retarded migration of circular molecules which makes it difficult to study circRNAs longer than ~600 nt in length.

1. Incubate 5 µg RNA in 50 mM $NaHCO_3$, pH 9 for 3 min at 90 °C. Include two control samples where the $NaHCO_3$ or the incubation is omitted (Table 4) (*see* **Note 11**).

2. Precipitate RNA (*see* Subheading 3.5).

3. Add 40 µL Urea Load Buffer to RNA pellet and re-suspend.

4. Incubate RNA for 30 s at 95 °C.

5. Load RNA on 6% PAGE (*see* Subheading 3.7).

Table 4
Alkaline hydrolysis of RNA

	Pos. (µL)	Neg.1 (µL)	Neg.2 (µL)
100 mM NaHCO$_3$, pH 9	25	25	0
H$_2$O	20	20	45
RNA (1 µg/µL)	5	5	5
Incubate for 3 min	90 °C	Ice	90 °C

3.5 RNA Precipitation

1. Add H$_2$O to adjust total volume of sample to 90 µL.
2. Then add 10 µL 3 M NaOAc, 250 µL 96% ethanol, and 0.5 µL glycogen (*see* **Note 12**).
3. Vortex the samples vigorously for 10–20 s.
4. Freeze on dry ice for 1 h.
5. Centrifuge >12,000 × g, at 4 °C for 30 min.
6. Decant the supernatant and add 1 mL 75% ethanol.
7. Centrifuge >12,000 × g, at 4 °C for 10 min.
8. Carefully remove the supernatant and all the residual ethanol (*see* **Notes 13** and **14**), and leave tube open to dry the pellet for approximately 5 min.

3.6 Agarose Gel Electrophoresis

The following steps applies to a ~10×10 cm agarose gel, scale accordingly to the relevant gel-dimensions. After gel-electrophoreses, the transfer of RNA described here is conducted by passive upward elution; however downward elution setups can also be used. The **steps 2–8** should be carried out in the fume hood:

1. Boil 1.2 g agarose in 89 mL H$_2$O.
2. In the fume hood, before casting the gel, allow the melted agarose to cool below 65 °C, and then add 2 mL 50× MOPS and 9 mL 37% formaldehyde. Then cast the gel.
3. While the gel solidifies, mix 10 µL RNA (1 g/L) with 20 µL Formamide Loading Buffer.
4. Remove comb and submerge gel in electrophoresis tank containing 1× MOPS running buffer. The gel should be completely covered with running buffer.
5. Prerun gel for 5 min, 75 V.
6. At the same time, denature RNA in loading buffer by incubating 5 min at 65 °C.
7. Load samples and run gel for ~3 h at 75 V.

8. After electrophoresis, wash the gel briefly in H_2O for 2 min.

9. Optional: Obtain an UV image of rRNA migration in a UV gel image system.

10. Wash the gel twice in 10× SSC for 20 min at room temperature.

11. While washing the gel, prepare two long sheets of 3 MM paper just slightly wider than the gel (here ~12 × 46 cm), three gel-sized 3 MM papers, and several layers of table paper.

12. Prepare a large tray with 10× SSC (~500 mL) with a glass plate on top.

13. Soak the two long sheets of 3 MM and place them over the glass plate with both ends in contact with the 10× SSC in the tray.

14. Place the gel upside-down on top of the 3 MM papers (*see* **Note 15**).

15. Briefly pre-wet a 10 × 10 cm Hybond™ N+ membrane in H_2O, then equilibrate in 10× SSC and place on top of gel (*see* **Note 15**).

16. Pre-soak the three 3 MM papers individually and add on top of the stack (*see* **Note 15**).

17. Place the layers of table paper, then a glass plate, and finally a ~500 g object (typically a bottle with ~500 mL H_2O) on top.

18. If possible, move to cold room and leave overnight.

19. The next day, continue with Subheading 3.8.

3.7 **PAGE**

The following description assumes a 3-mm thick gel sized 17 × 20 cm. Solutions can be scaled up or down for different gel dimensions. In contrast to the agarose gel, transfer from polyacrylamide gels requires electro-blotting instead of passive transfer.

1. First clean plates, spacers, and comb thoroughly with 10% SDS followed by 70% ethanol. Assemble the plates with the side and bottom-spacers in-between and fasten tightly with clamps.

2. Prepare the acrylamide solution (6% polyacrylamide gel, Table 5).

3. Pour the acrylamide solution carefully, place the comb, and wait 30–60 min (*see* **Note 16**).

4. After polymerization remove the clamps, the bottom spacer, and the comb. Attach the gel to a vertical electrophoresis apparatus and fill top and bottom compartments with 1× TBE. Wash the wells and the bottom of the gel with a syringe to remove bubbles, urea, and acrylamide debris. Prerun the gel for 1 h at 12 W at room temperature.

Table 5
Composition of a 50 mL, 6% PAGE

12 mL	SequaGel—UreaGel concentrate
33 mL	SequaGel—UreaGel diluent
5 mL	10× TBE
400 μL	10% APS
20 μL	TEMED

5. To prepare the RNA samples, mix the precipitated RNA pellet (*see* Subheading 3.5) with 40 μL Urea loading buffer (*see* **Note 17**).

6. Denature the RNA by heating the samples for 2 min at 95 °C.

7. While denaturing the RNA, wash the wells once again with a syringe.

8. Load the samples and run gel at 12 W for approximately 2 h. Bromophenol blue dye should reach the bottom of a gel.

9. After electrophoresis, move electrophoresis apparatus to the sink and dismount the gel.

10. Carefully separate the two glass plates and be aware of the gel orientation. It is recommended to mark the upper right corner of the acrylamide gel.

11. Fill tray with ethidium bromide stain and detach gel from glass plate in the solution. (*see* **Notes 16** and **18**).

12. Stain the gel for 20 min and obtain UV image of RNA migration and integrity.

13. Remove ethidium stain (this can be reused—store at 4 °C and avoid direct light exposure).

14. Fill tray with 0.5× TBE and wash the acrylamide gel for 30 min at room temperature.

15. Prepare six 3 MM papers and one Hybond™ N+ membrane the same size as the gel.

16. Pre-wet the membrane in H$_2$O.

17. To assemble the transfer, place individually three 3 MM papers pre-soaked in 0.5× TBE on one side of the transfer cassette.

18. Then carefully place the gel (*see* **Note 18**).

19. Equilibrate the membrane in 0.5× TBE and place it on top of the gel (*see* **Note 15**).

20. Place the remaining three 3 MM papers pre-soaked in 0.5× TBE.

21. Finally place a pre-soaked foam-pad on top and close the cassette.

22. Load the cassette into the Trans-blot apparatus. Be careful to position the cassette correctly (RNA is negatively charged).

23. Fill the Trans-blot chamber with 0.5× TBE and transfer overnight at 15 V at 4 °C. If possible, keep the Trans-blot on a magnetic stirrer to circulate the buffer.

3.8 Crosslinking Membrane

1. The membrane is carefully removed from the transfer setup. Mark the wells and the top-right corner to allow proper orientation of the membrane in the following steps.

2. Wash the membrane gently in 5× SSC to remove excess salt and gel remnants.

3. While lying on 3 MM paper, the membrane is UV crosslinked on both sides using 120 mJ/cm².

4. The membrane can now be stored for several months in a plastic wrap at 4 °C.

3.9 Hybridize Membrane

3.9.1 Label Probe

1. To radioactively label the DNA probe, mix 2.5 μL Probe (10 μM) with 13.5 μL H₂O (*see* **Notes 19–21**).

2. Incubate at 95 °C for 30 s, then cool solution instantly on ice.

3. Add 2 μL 10× Reaction Buffer A, 1 μL T4 Polynucleotide Kinase, and 1 μL [γ-32P]ATP. Incubate at 37 °C for 1 h.

4. After the incubation, add 30 μL H₂O to reaction mix and purify probe on G-50 column.

5. Measure the radioactivity on a Geiger counter. The probe should be >2000 counts per second at ~5 cm distance.

6. Store until use at −20 °C.

3.9.2 Hybridize Membrane

1. Pre-heat Church Buffer on a hot plate while stirring (at room-temperature, the SDS precipitates).

2. Place the membrane in a hybridization tube. Be sure that the RNA-side (facing the gel during transfer) is facing inward.

3. Pre-hybridize the membrane by adding 20 mL pre-heated Church Buffer to tube and incubate while rotating in hybridization oven at 55 °C for at least 30 min (*see* **Note 22**).

4. To prepare the hybridization buffer, boil the radioactively labeled probe for 1 min and mix with 20 mL pre-heated Church Buffer.

5. Discard the pre-hybridization buffer (the buffer is re-useable), and add the hybridization buffer containing the labeled probe.

6. Incubate overnight at 55 °C while rotating in the hybridization oven (*see* **Note 22**).

3.9.3 Wash and Expose Membrane

1. Discard the hybridization buffer (*see* **Notes 20** and **23**).

2. Wash membrane twice by adding 20 mL Washing Solution #1 and incubate while rotating at 50 °C for 15 min (*see* **Note 22**).

3. Optional, in case on high background noise, carry out one or two additional washes in Washing Solution #2 (*see* **Note 24**).

4. Remove the membrane from the hybridization tube and briefly wash membrane in Washing Solution #1 at room temperature. Place membrane on 3 MM paper to remove excess buffer (be careful not to dry membrane completely—it should remain moist).

5. Wrap membrane in plastic bag and expose in phosphor-imager cassette for 5 min to overnight depending on the signal, and process the cassette according to the manufacturer's instructions.

3.9.4 Stripping Membrane and Re-probing

1. To strip off the probe from the membrane, boil 100 mL Stripping Solution in the microwave oven.

2. Place the membrane in a plastic tray and pour the boiling solution onto the membrane.

3. Measure the signal with the Geiger-Müller counter and repeat stripping if signal persists.

4. Resume probing by pre-hybridizing membrane in pre-heated Church buffer as described above (from Subheading 3.9.2, **step 3**).

4   Notes

1. Here we use TRIzol® Reagent according to standard total RNA isolation protocols; however other commercially available total RNA purification kits can also be used. High RNA quality is vital and the methods described are not suitable for, e.g., FFPE-derived RNA.

2. We typically recommend using 60 nt probes with approximately 50% GC contents, although the probes used here varies in length. The probes should be blasted against the genome to avoid unspecific annealing. Using long probes (>100 nt) will presumably increase specificity; however they are very difficult to strip off the membrane.

3. Northern blotting is rather time consuming compared to other RNA detection techniques. However, several different experiments can be combined on the same northern membrane, and then prior to hybridization, the membrane is cut into distinct pieces comprising the individual experiments. Here, keep an empty well between experiments to ease the membrane separation.

4. Here, we use a rather low RNase R concentration (2 U/μg RNA) and short incubation (10 min) which is sufficient for northern blotting visualization, but it could be beneficial to use a higher concentration or extend the incubation period if qRT-PCR or RNA sequencing is the downstream choice of analysis. Partial trimming of linear RNA is clearly observed by northern blotting, but the 5′ region of linear RNA and internally structured RNA elements could in some cases exhibit partial RNase R resistance under reduced RNase levels and thereby could be mis-read using qRT-PCR as a circular RNA. Therefore, we recommend using 20 U/μg RNA for qRT-PCR analyses.

5. When analyzing transiently expressed RNA, it is important to include RNA from cells transfected with an empty vector (EV) to accurately distinguish specific from nonspecific signal.

6. We typically use Ribolock or other RNase inhibitors when incubating RNA at 37 °C to avoid unspecific RNase activity. Make sure that the RNase inhibitor used is not affecting RNase R or H.

7. When several samples are prepared in parallel, always to the extent possible prepare reactions as master mix to reduce variation between samples.

8. RNase R is known to require an unstructured 3'end to effectively trim and degrade the RNA substrate. Denaturing samples prior to incubation is therefore recommended.

9. It is important to include a negative control (without enzyme) but undergoing the exact same procedures to demarcate unspecific degradation from RNase R-mediated digestion.

10. The reaction volume could easily be scaled up if larger amounts of RNA are being treated. Using a 10 μL reaction volume, as described here, allows immediate loading of samples on northern without RNA precipitation.

11. We have tried the setup using 10–100 mM of final $NaHCO_3$ with similar effect (here 50 mM is used). Also, incubation from 2–6 min is suitable (here 3 min is used); however extended incubation leads to hyper-nicking (more than one nick per RNA) and a smeared result.

12. Glycogen is optional and only required for precipitating low quantify samples to produce a visible pellet. We typically use glycogen when precipitating below 10 μg.

13. After removal of the 75% ethanol used to wash the pellet during RNA precipitation, it is recommended to centrifuge the samples once again for 30 s to collect all the remaining ethanol at the bottom of the tube to aspirate with pipette.

14. When precipitating samples it is important to remove all residual ethanol as it may cause the samples to float out of the well

during loading of gel. However, over-drying the pellet may result in difficulties re-suspending RNA in loading buffer.

15. Air-bubbles impede the transfer of RNA to the membrane and should be removed. For example, use a 10 mL pipette to "roll out" any bubbles and repeat after applying each layer.

16. When working with hazardous solutions (such as acrylamide and ethidium bromide) wear appropriate gloves and protection, and always discard gloves immediately after handling the solutions to avoid contamination.

17. On the PAGE, it is possible to load at least 30 μg RNA in 40 μL Urea Loading Buffer.

18. When staining and washing a PAGE gel in a tray, it is recommended to keep a glass plate below the gel for better handling.

19. Northern blotting is not a very sensitive approach and should only be used on abundant RNA species—either highly abundant endogenous RNA or transiently expressed RNA. Combining multiple probes at once or using other detection strategies such as DIG-labeled oligos could enhance signal and sensitivity.

20. When working with radioactivity carefully follow the guidelines at your institution and always survey bench with Geiger-Müller counter for radioactive contamination afterward.

21. Probe the northern membrane for the lowest expressed RNA first and then re-probe for higher expressed RNA species afterward. Continuous stripping and re-probing will reduce the signal (we have successfully re-probed membrane 4 times without detrimental signal-loss). Also, even by extensive stripping, high signal bands (such as 18S) are very difficult to remove completely.

22. The temperatures used for hybridization and the subsequent washing steps depend on the melting temperature of the probe. We typically wash the membrane 5–10 °C below the hybridization temperature.

23. If you plan to use the probe again anytime soon, it is re-useable, however typically less effective in a second hybridization.

24. The membrane can always be subjected to additional wash-steps after exposure, but re-probing the membrane is considerably more work.

Acknowledgments

This work was supported by the Novo Nordisk Foundation (NNF16OC0019874).

References

1. Ebbesen KK, Kjems J, Hansen TB (2016) Circular RNAs: identification, biogenesis and function. Biochim Biophys Acta 1859:163–168

2. Hansen TB, Jensen TI, Clausen BH, Bramsen JB, Finsen B, Damgaard CK, Kjems J (2013) Natural RNA circles function as efficient microRNA sponges. Nature 495:384–388

3. Memczak S, Jens M, Elefsinioti A, Torti F, Krueger J, Rybak A, Maier L, Mackowiak SD, Gregersen LH, Munschauer M et al (2013) Circular RNAs are a large class of animal RNAs with regulatory potency. Nature 495:333–338

4. Zheng Q, Bao C, Guo W, Li S, Chen J, Chen B, Luo Y, Lyu D, Li Y, Shi G et al (2016) Circular RNA profiling reveals an abundant circHIPK3 that regulates cell growth by sponging multiple miRNAs. Nat Commun 7:11215

5. Ashwal-Fluss R, Meyer M, Pamudurti NR, Ivanov A, Bartok O, Hanan M, Evantal N, Memczak S, Rajewsky N, Kadener S (2014) circRNA biogenesis competes with pre-mRNA splicing. Mol Cell 56:55–66

6. Du WW, Yang W, Liu E, Yang Z, Dhaliwal P, Yang BB (2016) Foxo3 circular RNA retards cell cycle progression via forming ternary complexes with p21 and CDK2. Nucleic Acids Res 44:2846–2858

7. Jeck WR, Sorrentino JA, Wang K, Slevin MK, Burd CE, Liu J, Marzluff WF, Sharpless NE (2012) Circular RNAs are abundant, conserved, and associated with ALU repeats. RNA 19(2):141–152

8. Zhang XO, Wang HB, Zhang Y, Lu X, Chen LL, Yang L (2014) Complementary sequence-mediated exon circularization. Cell 159:134–147

9. Liang D, Wilusz JE (2014) Short intronic repeat sequences facilitate circular RNA production. Genes Dev 28:2233–2247

10. Dong R, Ma XK, Chen LL, Yang L (2016) Increased complexity of circRNA expression during species evolution. RNA Biol:1–11

11. Rybak-Wolf A, Stottmeister C, Glazar P, Jens M, Pino N, Giusti S, Hanan M, Behm M, Bartok O, Ashwal-Fluss R et al (2015) Circular RNAs in the mammalian brain are highly abundant, conserved, and dynamically expressed. Mol Cell 58:870–885

12. Wang PL, Bao Y, Yee MC, Barrett SP, Hogan GJ, Olsen MN, Dinneny JR, Brown PO, Salzman J (2014) Circular RNA is expressed across the eukaryotic tree of life. PLoS One 9:e90859

13. Veno MT, Hansen TB, Veno ST, Clausen BH, Grebing M, Finsen B, Holm IE, Kjems J (2015) Spatio-temporal regulation of circular RNA expression during porcine embryonic brain development. Genome Biol 16:245

14. Houseley J, Tollervey D (2010) Apparent non-canonical trans-splicing is generated by reverse transcriptase in vitro. PLoS One 5:e12271

15. You X, Vlatkovic I, Babic A, Will T, Epstein I, Tushev G, Akbalik G, Wang M, Glock C, Quedenau C et al (2015) Neural circular RNAs are derived from synaptic genes and regulated by development and plasticity. Nat Neurosci 18:603–610

16. Barrett SP, Wang PL, Salzman J (2015) Circular RNA biogenesis can proceed through an exon-containing lariat precursor. elife 4:e07540

17. Suzuki H, Zuo Y, Wang J, Zhang MQ, Malhotra A, Mayeda A (2006) Characterization of RNase R-digested cellular RNA source that consists of lariat and circular RNAs from pre-mRNA splicing. Nucleic Acids Res 34:e63

18. Suzuki H, Tsukahara T (2014) A view of pre-mRNA splicing from RNase R resistant RNAs. Int J Mol Sci 15:9331–9342

19. Capel B, Swain A, Nicolis S, Hacker A, Walter M, Koopman P, Goodfellow P, Lovell-Badge R (1993) Circular transcripts of the testis-determining gene Sry in adult mouse testis. Cell 73:1019–1030

20. Pasman Z, Been MD, Garcia-Blanco MA (1996) Exon circularization in mammalian nuclear extracts. RNA 2:603–610

21. Ruskin B, Krainer AR, Maniatis T, Green MR (1984) Excision of an intact intron as a novel lariat structure during pre-mRNA splicing in vitro. Cell 38:317–331

Chapter 13

Characterization of Circular RNAs (circRNA) Associated with the Translation Machinery

Deniz Bartsch, Anne Zirkel, and Leo Kurian

Abstract

A substantial proportion of the currently annotated genes in eukaryotes are proposed to function as RNA molecules (>200 bp) with no significant protein coding potential, currently classified as long noncoding RNAs (lncRNA). A distinct subgroup of lncRNAs is circular RNAs (circRNAs), which can be easily identified by unique junction reads, resulting from their biogenesis. CircRNAs are largely cytosolic and thought to either code for micro-peptides or facilitate gene regulation by sequestering microRNAs (miRNAs) or RNA-binding proteins (RBPs) from their targets. Interrogation of the interaction of circRNAs with cellular macromolecular machineries could indicate their mode of action. Here, we detail a sucrose gradient-based method to pinpoint association of a given circRNA (or any transcript of interest) with distinct ribosomal fractions. This method can evaluate the coding potential of candidate circRNAs (or any transcript of interest) and its association with the translation machinery.

Key words circRNA, Polysome profiling, Ribosome profiling, circRNA detection by RT-qPCR - Protein-coding potential by polysome profiling

1 Introduction

The advent of massively parallel sequencing methods led to the discovery of a vast number of long noncoding RNA (lncRNA) transcripts in eukaryotes, which were long classified as transcriptional noise [1]. Further studies demonstrated a diverse spectrum of biological functions for these versatile molecules, ranging from epigenetic modulation to translational regulation [2]. A subgroup of these lncRNAs termed circRNAs have recently gained focus partly due to its unique molecular organization and tissue-specificity [3, 4]. CircRNAs are formed by back-splicing of pre-mRNAs leading to the formation of a circular transcript (Fig. 1), which can be monoexonic, multi-exonic or even contain intronic regions [5, 6]. They have been reported to regulate myriad processes including transcription, splicing [7] and translation by sequestering RNA-binding proteins or miRNAs (functioning as

Christoph Dieterich and Argyris Papantonis (eds.), *Circular RNAs: Methods and Protocols*, Methods in Molecular Biology, vol. 1724, https://doi.org/10.1007/978-1-4939-7562-4_13, © Springer Science+Business Media, LLC 2018

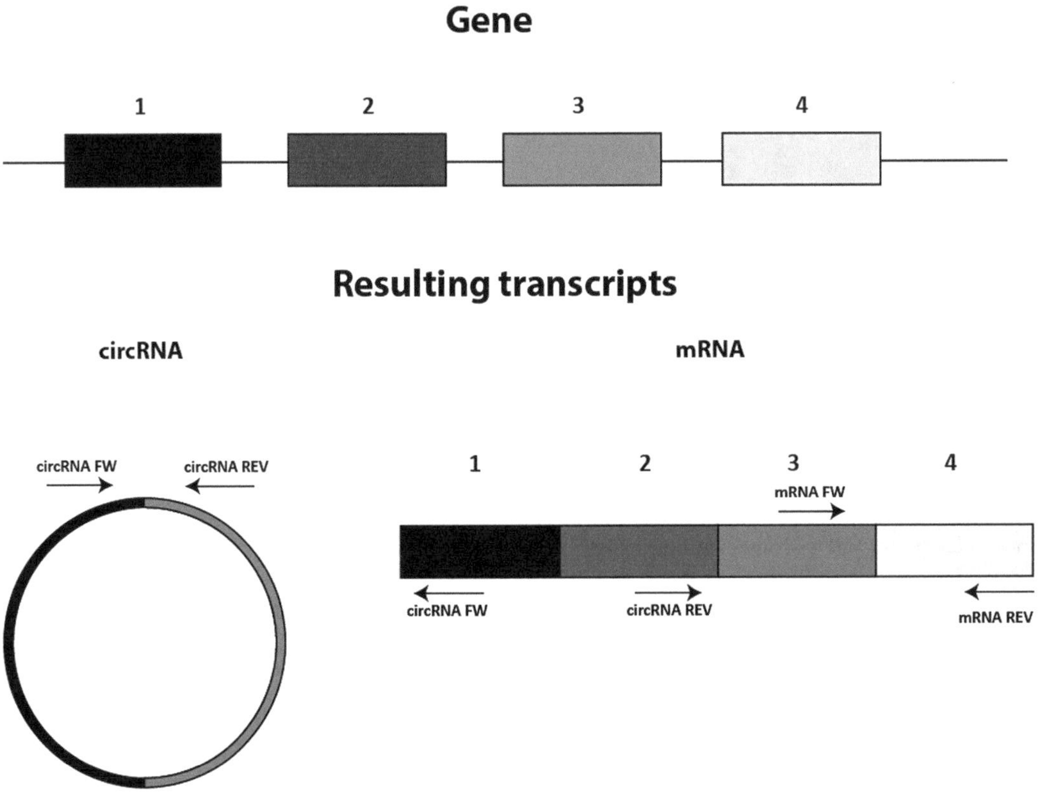

Gene

Fig. 1 Illustration of a qPCR based strategy to specifically distinguish circRNAs from cognate mRNAs. CircRNAs originate from back-splicing events resulting in unique junctions, which can be used as target sequences for primers. In the depicted example, circRNA-specific primers only yield a PCR product from circRNAs due to the backsplicing event leading to circularization, while in a regular mRNA both of these primers would face opposite directions. On contrary, mRNA specific primers binding to regions not present in the circRNA (e.g. untranslated regions (UTRs) or specific exonic regions) can be used to distinctly detect the cognate mRNA

miRNA sponges) from their targets [2, 8]. Emerging evidence indicates that some of them can code for functional micro-peptides. Here we demonstrate a protocol to investigate the association of candidate circRNAs with distinct fractions of translation machinery, which enables to assess their coding potential or a possible role in translational regulation. This method is adapted from sucrose density gradient fractionation of cellular lysates. Tracing the RNA content via UV absorption at 254 nm results in a characteristic translational profile [9, 10]. This fractionation enables the separation of cytosolic RNAs (not associated with ribosomes) or RNA molecules associated with 40S ribosomal subunit, 60S ribosomal subunit, monosomes (80S), and polysomes (Fig. 2). RNA isolated from aforementioned fractions can be subjected to RT-qPCR to measure the enrichment of a candidate RNA in either of the fractions in a quantitative manner. Additionally, we provide evidence for the feasibility of this method

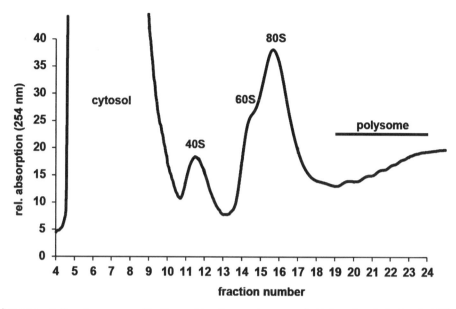

Fig. 2 A representative ribosome profile. The cell lysates can be separated into cytosolic (cytosol), 40S subunit, 60S subunit, 80S (monosome) and polysomes fractions, after separation via sucrose gradient centrifugation

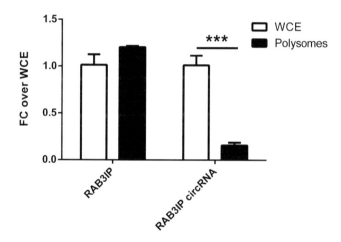

Fig. 3 RAB3IP circRNA is not associated with the translational machinery, a proof of principle study. A qPCR-based evaluation for the association of RAB3IP circRNA and its cognate mRNA with the translational machinery. After normalizing to the whole cell (WCE) extract levels, the data indicates that RAB3IB circRNA is not associated with the translational machinery, while the cognate mRNA is bound by polysomes

using a gene that encodes both an mRNA and a circRNA. Our data demonstrate that the mRNA transcript is enriched in the polysome fractions, while the cognate circRNA is significantly de-enriched (Fig. 3).

2   Materials

Prepare all solutions using DNase-free/RNase-free water (*see* **Note 1**). All solutions are stored at 4 °C and kept on ice while in use unless indicated otherwise. We strongly recommend working in a sterile and RNase-free environment.

1. Ribosome profiling buffer: Mix 20 mM Tris, 150 mM NaCl, and 5 mM $MgCl_2$ in water and adjust pH to 7.4 with HCl. Add 1% Triton X-100 from 20% Triton X-100 stock. Store at RT. Prior to usage add 1 mM DTT, 100 µg/mL cycloheximide, RNase-Inhibitor, and EDTA-free protease inhibitor and keep on ice (*see* **Notes 1–3**).

2. Sucrose gradient buffer: Mix 20 mM Tris, 140 mM KCl, and 1.5 mM $MgCl_2$ in water and adjust pH to 7.8 with HCl. Prior to usage add 1 mM DTT, 100 µg/mL cycloheximide, RNase-Inhibitor, and EDTA-free protease inhibitor and keep on ice.

3. Sucrose gradient solutions: For 10 and 50% sucrose solutions dissolve 10 g/50 g sucrose in 100 mL sucrose gradient buffer, sterile filter, and store at 4 °C.

4. Fractionation solution: Dissolve 70 g sucrose in RNAse-free water, sterile filter, and store at RT.

5. Ice bucket.

6. RNaseZap® (Life Technologies, Darmstadt, Germany) or comparable RNase decontaminant solution.

7. Ethanol 70% (v/v).

8. Gradient maker (BioComp Instruments, Fredericton, Canada).

9. Thin-wall polypropylene tubes.

10. SW-41 Ti Rotor and Optima™ XE centrifuge (Beckman Coulter, Krefeld, Germany), or comparable ultracentrifuge.

11. Foxy R2 fraction collector, Tris peristaltic pump DFS, UA-6 detector W Type 11 (Teledyne Isco, Lincoln, USA).

12. TRIzol® Reagent (Life Technologies, Darmstadt, Germany) or a comparable phenol/chloroform-based RNA isolation reagent.

13. Chloroform.

14. 2-Propanol.

15. 70% Ethanol.

16. Reverse transcription mix (1 reaction): 5 µL 5× RT buffer, 0.5 µL 100 mM dNTPs, 1 µL, 0.1 µg/µL random hexamer primers, 0.1 µL reverse transcriptase, 3.4 µL H_2O.

17. SYBR green qPCR (Bio-Rad Laboratories, Munich, Germany) or comparable qPCR mix.

18. CFX96 Touch™ Real-Time PCR Detection System (Bio-Rad Laboratories, Munich, Germany).

3   Methods

3.1   Harvesting Cell Culture Samples

Carry out all procedures at room temperature in RNase-free environment unless otherwise specified.

1. Grow desired cell type to around 80% density (*see* **Note 5**).
2. Add 100 μg/mL cycloheximide to the culture medium and incubate for 5 min at 37 °C and 5% CO_2.
3. Wash once with ice-cold DPBS containing 100 μg/mL cycloheximide.
4. Scrape down cells with a sterile cell dispenser using ice-cold PBS, spin down at 300 × g for 2 min at 4 °C, discard the supernatant, and directly snap freeze the pellet (*see* **Note 6**).
5. Store pellets at −80 °C until further usage.

3.2   Cell Lysis

1. Resuspend the cell pellet 1 mL of pre-chilled ribosome profiling buffer and incubate on ice for 10 min.
2. Triturate the suspension with a sterile 27-G needle ten times and centrifuge for 10 min at 20,000 × g and 4 °C.
3. Transfer the supernatant to a fresh microcentrifuge tube and store on ice until sucrose gradient (*see* Subheading 3.3).
4. Mix 100 μL lysate with 500 μL Trizol and store at −80 °C as input RNA sample (*see* **Note 6**).

3.3   Preparing the Continuous 10–50% Sucrose Gradient

1. Mark the conical ultracentrifuge tubes with an ethanol-proof marker.
2. Fill until the marker line with the 10% sucrose solution by using a pipette.
3. With a sterile syringe carefully add the 50% sucrose solution below the 10% sucrose solution.
4. Seal the tubes with long caps and remove excess sucrose solution.
5. Carefully transfer the tubes into the magnetic rack and prepare continuous 10–50% sucrose gradients with a gradient maker.
6. Remove 500 μL of the prepared gradient and add the lysates. Balance the tubes using polysome buffer (*see* **Note 7**). Transfer the centrifugation tubes to the rotor buckets and store at 4 ° C.

3.4   Sucrose Gradient Fractionation

1. Precool the ultracentrifuge to 4 ° C prior to preparing the gradients.
2. Put the rotor tubes in the rotor and transfer it to the ultracentrifuge.
3. Centrifuge the samples for 3 h at 2,60,000 × g and 4 °C using minimal acceleration and deceleration.

4. After centrifugation put the rotor buckets on ice.

5. Assemble fraction collector and tubings of the peristaltic pump.

6. Attach an empty centrifugation tube to the fraction collector and wash the tubings once by pumping autoclaved water, followed by one wash with 70% ethanol.

7. Equilibrate the tubings by pumping with 70% sucrose solution until it reaches the tip of the needle (*see* **Note 8**).

8. Remove the centrifugation tube used for washing and attach the sample centrifugation tube to the fractionator.

9. Push the needle through the bottom of the tube.

10. Start fractionation by pumping with 70% sucrose solution with a speed of 1 mL/min.

11. Record the UV absorption at 254 nm and identify specific fractions.

12. Collect fractions corresponding to cytosol, 40S, 60S, 80S, and polysomes (*see* Fig. 2, **Note 9**).

3.5 RNA Isolation and RT-qPCR

1. Add 1 mL Trizol to the collected fractions for RNA isolation (*see* **Notes 6** and **10**).

2. Isolate RNA from collected fractions according to the manufacturer's protocol.

3. Add 1 μg of RNA (in a total amount of 15 μL) to 10 μL RT master mix.

4. Incubate for 10 min at 21 °C.

5. Incubate for 60 min at 42 °C.

6. Deactivate the enzyme by heat shock for 10 min at 65 °C.

7. Dilute the cDNA in 175 μL water.

8. Use 2 μL cDNA as template for the qPCR.

9. Add 2.5 qPCR master mix and 0.5 μL 10 μM forward and reverse primer mix (*see* **Notes 11** and **12**).

4 Notes

1. We use deionized water, which was treated with diethyl pyrocarbonate (DEPC) for 12 h and followed by autoclaving.

2. Cycloheximide and other translation inhibitors can result in ribosomal occupancy biases across the length of an RNA molecule. This should be taken into account while data analysis [11].

3. We use RNase Inhibitor, Murine (NEB, Ipswich, USA). 10 μL per in 1 mL of lysate is recommended, but varies between cell types depending on endogenous RNase levels.

4. Using ethylenediaminetetraacetic acid (EDTA) causes ribosome disassembly and results in bad profiles and thus should be avoided.

5. We used human umbilical endothelial cells (HUVECs). The number of cells required for a good polysome profile depends on the cell type of interest and needs to be evaluated. Generally, overgrowing cells reduces translation rates and should be avoided if not subject of the investigation.

6. Cell pellets can be stored at −80 °C for up to a month without affecting the efficiency of the protocol.

7. Balancing should be as precise as possible. Samples should not vary more than 0.001 g.

8. While washing and equilibrating the tubings any air bubble needs to be removed. Air bubbles disturb the gradient and thus result in bad profiles.

9. The appearance of a polysome profile may vary depending on cell type and organism of interest. Based on the translational output of given cell type, different profile peaks can be more or less pronounced.

10. We recommend adding spike-in controls to improve the reliability of qPCRs. Suitable controls are bacterial mRNAs not expressed in the investigated cell type, as well as GFP or luciferase mRNA, which can be added to the fractions after fraction collection, to rule out any RNA purification bias.

11. Primers should be designed for circRNA-specific sequences, flanking the junction created by back splicing (Fig. 1). Cognate mRNA transcripts can be distinguished by using primers binding mRNA-specific regions like the 3′ UTR.

12. Additionally, 18S and 28 rRNA primers can serve as internal controls. Both rRNAs should be de-enriched in the cytoplasmic fraction. 18S should be enriched in the 40S fraction and 28S should be enriched in the 60S. Both rRNAs together should be increasing from 80S to heavy polysomal fractions.

Acknowledgments

The Kurian lab is supported by the NRW Stem Cell Network Independent Group Leader Grant, CECAD, German Heart Association (DZHK), Else Kröner Fresenius-Stiftung (Grant No. 3640 0626 21) and University of Cologne (Grant No: 3681000801 and 2681101801). We would like to thank Prof. Elena Rugarli and CECAD, Cologne, for access to the polysome fractionator.

References

1. Iyer MK, Niknafs YS, Malik R et al (2015) The landscape of long noncoding RNAs in the human transcriptome. Nat Genet 47:199–208. https://doi.org/10.1038/ng.3192
2. Mercer T, Dinger M, Mattick J (2009) Long non-coding RNAs: insights into functions. Nat Rev Genet 10:155–159
3. Memczak S, Jens M, Elefsinioti A et al (2013) Circular RNAs are a large class of animal RNAs with regulatory potency. Nature 495:333–338. https://doi.org/10.1038/nature11928
4. Guo JU, Agarwal V, Guo H, Bartel DP (2014) Expanded identification and characterization of mammalian circular RNAs. Genome Biol 15:409. https://doi.org/10.1186/PREACCEPT-1176565312639289
5. Wang Y, Wang Z (2015) Efficient backsplicing produces translatable circular mRNAs. RNA 21:172–179. https://doi.org/10.1261/rna.048272.114
6. Barrett SP, Wang PL, Salzman J (2015) Circular RNA biogenesis can proceed through an exon-containing lariat precursor. Elife 4:e07540. https://doi.org/10.7554/eLife.07540
7. Zlotorynski E (2015) Non-coding RNA: circular RNAs promote transcription. Nat Rev Mol Cell Biol 16:3967. https://doi.org/10.1038/nrm3967
8. Toit a D (2013) RNA: circular RNAs as miRNA sponges. Nat Rev Mol Cell Biol 14:11993. https://doi.org/10.1038/nrm3557
9. Lazarides EL, Lukens LN, Infante AA (1971) Collagen polysomes: site of hydroxylation of proline residues. J Mol Biol 58:831–846. https://doi.org/10.1016/0022-2836(71)90043-X
10. Rivera MC, Maguire B, Lake JA (2015) Purification of polysomes. Cold Spring Harb Protoc 2015:303–305. https://doi.org/10.1101/pdb.prot081364
11. Gerashchenko MV, Gladyshev VN (2014) Translation inhibitors cause abnormalities in ribosome profiling experiments. Nucleic Acids Res 42:e134. https://doi.org/10.1093/nar/gku671

Chapter 14

Synthesis and Engineering of Circular RNAs

Sonja Petkovic and Sabine Müller

Abstract

Circular RNAs (circRNAs) have been discovered in all kingdoms of life. They are produced from introns as well as from exons. However, strongest interest is in circRNAs that are transcribed and spliced from exons of protein and noncoding genes in eukaryotic cells including humans. Therefore, synthesis and engineering of circRNAs as models for structure and function studies are strongly required. In vitro, methods for RNA synthesis and circularization are available. Chemical synthesis allows for preparation of RNAs incorporating nonnatural nucleotides in small RNA segments, whereas enzymatic synthesis is advantageous for production of long RNAs, however, without the possibility for site-specific modification. Strategies for chemical and enzymatic RNA synthesis may be combined to obtain long modified linear RNA strands for subsequent circularization. Here, we describe two alternative protocols for synthesis and circularization in dependence on downstream applications and template structure.

Key words Chemical synthesis, Ligation, Circularization, GMP-priming, In vitro transcription

1 Introduction

Circular RNAs (circRNAs) have been identified in all kingdoms of life, across species from Archaea to humans [1–5]. Their exact functions still remain largely speculative. However, first indications of specific roles are emerging [6]. The biogenesis of circRNAs is supposed to occur by noncanonical back splicing in alternative scenarios [7, 8]. For in vitro RNA circularization, ligation strategies adapted from procedures for intermolecular ligation by chemical, enzymatic, or DNAzyme-supported protocols are available [9]. Key issue of all procedures is the goal of obtaining a natural 3′,5′-linkage and to favor circularization over intermolecular end joining, which would lead to oligomerization. In addition to the formation of natural phosphodiester linkages, chemical strategies for circularization might profit from available powerful chemistries for end joining, which however would produce nonnatural linkages. Prior to circularization, linear RNA is prepared by either chemical synthesis or enzymatic transcription in vitro (Figs. 1 and 2). Chemical synthesis allows for fast and cheap generation of

Christoph Dieterich and Argyris Papantonis (eds.), *Circular RNAs: Methods and Protocols*, Methods in Molecular Biology, vol. 1724, https://doi.org/10.1007/978-1-4939-7562-4_14, © Springer Science+Business Media, LLC 2018

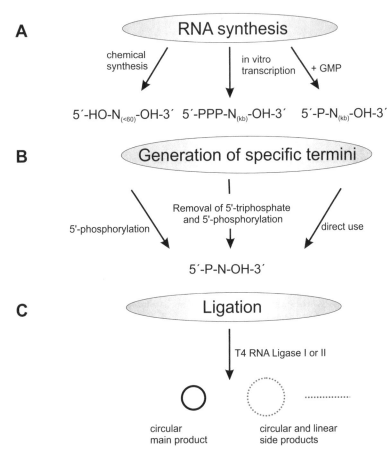

Fig. 1 Synthesis and circularization of RNA. Workflow composed of the three major steps: (**A**) RNA preparation by chemical synthesis (left) or enzymatic in vitro transcription (middle and right), eventually primed with GMP (right). (**B**) Generation of specific termini for ligation, in particular introduction of a 5′-monophosphate. Products of general in vitro transcription have to be dephosphorylated prior to 5′-rephosphorylation; products of GMP-primed in vitro transcription can be directly used. (**C**) Ligation with T4 RNA ligase I or II, dependent on the ligation junction positioned in a single- or double-stranded area of the substrate. Circular or linear oligomers can be formed as side products

RNAs of any backbone, base modifications, and linkages, and therefore gives access to a broad range of modified or specifically functionalized RNAs. As an alternative to chemical RNA synthesis, enzymatic protocols yield long RNAs that may have lengths in the kb range. However, the introduction of modified bases or alternative backbones is less straightforward, due to limited RNA polymerase substrate tolerance and impossibility of site-specific positioning. For the production of long modified circRNAs, chemically synthesized site-specifically modified RNA segments need to be ligated prior to or simultaneously with circularization.

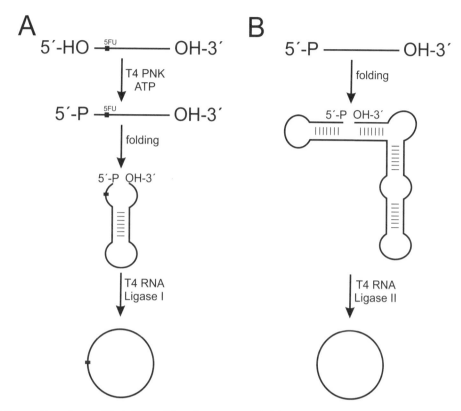

Fig. 2 Preparation of a modified 49mer (**A**) and a non-modified 83mer (**B**) circRNA as described in the protocols. (**A**) The linear precursor site-specifically modified with 5-fluorouridine (5FU) was chemically synthesized followed by 5'-phosphorylation with polynucleotide kinase (PNK). Under native conditions the RNA folds into a dumbbell-shaped structure with the ligation junction positioned in a single-stranded region. Circularization proceeds by ligation with T4 RNA ligase I. (**B**) The linear 5'-phosphorylated precursor was produced by in vitro transcription primed with GMP. Folding under native conditions positions the ligation junction in a double-stranded region. Circularization proceeds by ligation with T4 RNA ligase II

In vitro-transcribed RNAs carry a 5'-triphosphate and a 3'-hydroxyl group. Therefore, 5'-dephosphorylation is necessary prior to circularization, to initially generate RNA with hydroxyl groups at both termini (as for the chemical synthesis, Fig. 1).

Enzymatic ligation of RNA requires substrates with 5'-monophosphate and free 3'-hydroxyl group. Therefore, the 5'-OH group of chemically synthesized RNAs as well as of in vitro-transcribed and dephosphorylated RNAs has to be converted into a phosphomonoester. This can be achieved by enzymatic phosphorylation with polynucleotide kinase and ATP. As an alternative, the 5'-monophosphate can be directly produced during in vitro transcription by transcription priming with guanosine monophosphate (GMP) [10]. An excess of GMP over GTP and the other three nucleotides primes the nascent RNA with GMP as first nucleotide instead of GTP. Using this strategy, 70–90% of the RNAs may contain GMP [11] at the

5′-terminus, thus allowing direct use in ligation assays. It is even possible to use the transcription mixture straight for RNA circularization by T4 RNA ligase; only the GMP-primed RNA is accepted as substrate, whereas the triphosphorylated RNA (that is also still produced by in vitro transcription) is not. Alternatively, the GMP-primed RNA is first isolated from the in vitro transcription mixture, preferentially by electrophoresis through a polyacrylamide gel, and then circularized. For circularization mostly T4 RNA ligase is used. However, also specially designed ribozymes may be used as described elsewhere [10, 12].

The efficiency of ligation and in particular the preferred intramolecular reaction leading to circularization is highly dependent on the RNA structure. In order to suppress the most significant side reaction, which is intermolecular end joining leading to oligomerization, experimental design is most important. One option is to favor intramolecular ligation (circularization) over intermolecular ligation (oligomerization) by working at small concentrations of the linear precursor (Fig. 3). In addition, and probably more effectively, self-templating effects based on the intrinsic structure of the linear precursor can assist pre-orientation of the two ends to be linked in an intramolecular fashion. Alternatively, helper oligonucleotides may be included to achieve the desired pre-orientation of reacting ends [9]. Dependent on the ligation junction positioned in a single-stranded or a double-stranded area, T4 RNA ligase I or T4

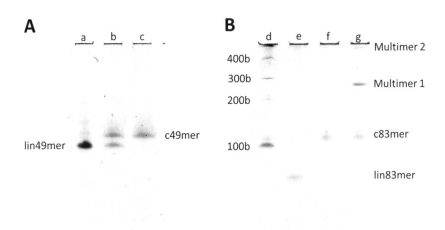

Fig. 3 Results of two different ligation protocols. (**A**) Circularization of a single-stranded 49mer RNA prepared by chemical synthesis (comp. Fig. 2A) with T4 RNA ligase I. Lane a: Linear 49mer as size control, b: 49mer circularized with a yield of ca. 50%, c: ligation mixture treated with RNase R according to 3.10. (**B**) Circularization of a single-stranded 83mer RNA prepared by GMP-primed in vitro transcription (comp. Fig. 2B) with T4 RNA ligase II. d: Commercial RNA size standard: RNA RiboRuler low-range RNA ladder, e: linear 83mer as size control, f: circularized 83mer (at 20 nM concentration of the linear precursor), g: circularized 83mer and multimeric side products (at 200 nM concentration of the linear precursor)

RNA ligase II is used, respectively. Both enzymes require ATP for activation of the phosphorylated RNA 5′-terminus as adenylate (AppRNA), and catalyze the nucleophilic attack of the 3′-OH terminus onto the activated 5′-terminus to form a covalent 5′, 3′-phosphodiester bond. As mentioned above, intermolecular end joining (oligomerization) is a serious side reaction, which cannot be completely suppressed. Isolation of the circular product from any oligomerized species can be achieved by electrophoresis through polyacrylamide gels, optionally in combination with hydrolysis of all linear species by RNase R prior to electrophoresis (Fig. 3).

Here we describe the chemical synthesis of a small RNA (49 nts) site-specifically modified with 5-fluorouridine followed by circularization with T4 RNA ligase I (Fig. 2A). Furthermore, we provide protocols for preparation of a 5′-phosphorylated RNA (83 nts) by in vitro transcription primed with GMP, and circularization with T4 RNA ligase II (Fig. 2B).

2 Materials

2.1 General Information

Chemicals were obtained from commercial suppliers (Merck, Sigma-Aldrich, Roth, Acros, Fluka, and VWR) and used without further purification unless otherwise noted. All buffers for PAGE and HPLC purification were filtered through a 0.2 μm membrane. All solutions for nucleic acid purification by PAGE were filtered and degassed using low pressure. All buffers used in RNA purification or reactions were prepared from autoclaved Millipore water with a resistivity of 18.2 M W/cm and were filtered as described above prior to use.

2.2 Apparatus

1. Gene Assembler Special, Pharmacia.
2. Äkta Purifier, Amersham Biosciences.
3. Anion-exchange column: DNAPac PA-100 22 × 50 mm, Guard and DNAPac PA-100 22 × 250 mm, PrepScale, Dionex, BioLC.
4. Reversed-phase column: VarioPrep Guard 50/10 Nucleodur 100-5C18ec and VarioPrep 250/10 Nucleodur 100-5C18ec, Macherey-Nagel.
5. Centrifuge 5804 R and 5804, Eppendorf.
6. UV transilluminator: Chemi Smart 2000, VilberLourmat.
7. NanoDrop ND-1000 Spectrophotometer, PeqLab.
8. Table centrifuge, Roth.
9. Thermoblock T Gradient, Biometra.
10. Typhoon FLA 9000, GE Healthcare Life Sciences.
11. Concentrator, Savant.
12. PAGE system, Hoefer, Pharmacia Biotech AB.

2.3 Chemical RNA Synthesis

1. Phosphoramidite building blocks: 5′-(4,4′-Dimethoxytrityl)-N-phenoxyacetyl-adenosine-2′-O-TBDMS-3′-[(2-cyanoethyl)-(N,N-diisopropyl)]-phosphoramidite (Link Technologies), 5′-(4,4′-dimethoxytrityl)-N-acetyl-cytidine-2′-O-TBDMS-3′-[(2-cyanoethyl)-(N,N-diisopropyl)]-phosphor-amidite (Link Technologies), 5′-(4,4′-dimethoxytrityl)-N-(4-isopropyl-phenoxyacetyl)-guanosine-2′-O-TBDMS-3′-[(2-cyanoethyl)-(N,N-diisopropyl)]-phosphoramidite (Link Technologies), 5′-(4,4′-dimethoxytrityl)-uridine-2′-O-TBDMS-3′-[(2-cyanoethyl)-(N,N-diisopropyl)]-phosphoramidite (Link Technologies), 5′-(4,4′-dimethoxytrityl)-5-fluorouridine-2′-O-TBDMS-3′-[(2-cyanoethyl)-(N,N-diisopropyl)]-phosphoramidite (ChemGenes).

2. Acetonitrile (99.9% extra dry over molecular sieves from ACROS or anhydrous with water content under 20 ppm from emp Biotech).

3. Solid-phase support as CPG (controlled pore glass) functionalized with A, C, G, and U: Pac-rASynBase, CPG 1000/110, 37 μmol/g (Link Technologies), Ac-rCSynbase, CPG 1000/110, 36 μmol/g (Link Technologies), iPr-Pac-rGSynbase, CPG 2.1. Variants1000/110, 23 μmol/g (Link Technologies), U RNA Synbase, CPG 1000/110, 44 μmol/g (Link Technologies)

4. Oxidation solution: 0.01 M Iodine, 260 mL acetonitrile (HPLC grade), 24 mL trimethylpyridine, 120 mL water.

5. Capping A: 20% N-methylimidazole in acetonitrile: 15.86 mL N-methylimidazole, 84.14 mL acetonitrile (HPLC grade).

6. Capping B: 50 mL Acetonitrile (HPLC grade), 20 mL acetic anhydride, 30 mL trimethylpyridine.

7. Detritylation: 970 mL 1,2-Dichloroethane, 30 mL dichloroacetic acid.

8. Activator: 0.3 M in acetonitrile: 2.3 g BMT (5-benzylmercaptotetrazole from emp Biotech) in 40 mL acetonitrile (99.9% extra dry over molecular sieves from ACROS or anhydrous with water content under 20 ppm from emp Biotech).

9. Molecular sieves for amidite solution and activator solution: 3 Ångström, activated (Roth).

2.4 Deprotection

1. Deprotection solution: 1:1 (v/v) mixture of 8 M ethanolic methylamine and concentrated NH_3 (30%).

2. Desilylation reagent: 3:1 (v/v) mixture of $NEt_3 \times 3$ HF and DMF (dry 99.8% ACROS Extra Dry over AcroSeal).

3. *n*-Butanol: Analytical grade.

4. TEAA buffer: 0.05 M Triethylammonium acetate, pH 7.0.

2.5 Purification of Chemically Synthesized RNA by Denaturing PAGE

1. TBE (1×): 0.1 M Tris, 1 mM EDTA, 85 mM boric acid, pH 8.3.

2. Gel solution: 20% Acrylamide/bisacrylamide 19:1 (Roth), 1× TBE, 7 M urea.

3. Ammonium persulfate: 10% Solution in water.

4. N,N,N',N'-tetramethylethylene diamine (TEMED).

5. Loading buffer: 98:2 (v/v) mixture of formamide and 0.5 M EDTA.

6. Eluting buffer: 0.5 M LiOAc.

2.6 Purification by Anion-Exchange HPLC

1. Columns named in Subheading 2.2.

2. Buffer A: 10 mM Tris, 10 mM $NaClO_4$, 6 M urea, pH 7.0.

3. Buffer B: 10 mM Tris, 500 mM $NaClO_4$, 6 M urea, pH 7.0.

2.7 RNA Precipitation

1. $MgCl_2$ (20 Vol%, 50 mM).

2. Sodium acetate (3 M, 10 Vol%, pH 5.3).

3. Ethanol (250 Vol%, analytical grade).

2.8 Ethanol/Acetone Precipitation

1. Ethanol analytical grade.

2. Acetone analytical grade.

2.9 RP Chromatography

1. Reversed-phase column (Sep-Pak Vac 12 cc (2 g), C18, Waters).

2. Acetonitrile (HPLC grade).

3. Triethylammonium bicarbonate buffer (100 mM, TBK buffer pH 8.5 Fluka).

4. Acetonitrile/water 3:2 (v/v).

2.10 Gel Filtration

1. Sephadex G25 fine (1 g, GE Healthcare).

2. Autoclaved millipore water.

2.11 In Vitro Transcription

1. HEPES buffer (1×): 50 mM HEPES-Na, 12 mM $MgCl_2$, 2 mM spermidine, 40 mM DTT, pH 7.5.

2. NTP mixture: Use a stock solution with 25 mM of each rNTP.

3. dsDNA template, e.g., Klenow or a DNA plasmid: 1 μM.

4. RiboLock: 40 U/μL (RNase free, Thermo Fisher Scientific).

5. T7 RNA polymerase: 20 U/mL (RNase free, Thermo Fisher Scientific).

6. DNase I: 2 U (RNase free, Thermo Fisher Scientific).

7. 250 Vol% ethanol abs.

2.12 In Vitro Transcription with GMP Priming

1. HEPES buffer (1×): 50 mM HEPES-Na, 12 mM $MgCl_2$, 2 mM spermidine, 40 mM DTT, pH 7.5.

2. rNTP mixture: ATP, CTP, UTP each 2 mM, GTP: 0.625 mM, GMP: 3 mM.

3. dsDNA template, e.g., Klenow or a DNA plasmid: 1 µM.

4. RiboLock: 40 U/µL (RNase free, Thermo Fisher Scientific).

5. T7 RNA polymerase: 20 U/mL (RNase free, Thermo Fisher Scientific).

6. DNase I: 2 U (RNase free, Thermo Fisher Scientific).

7. 250 Vol% ethanol abs.

2.13 Purification and/or Analysis by Denaturing PAGE

1. TBE buffer (10×), 0.89 M Tris–HCl, 0.89 M boric acid, 0.02 M EDTA-Na, pH 8.3. Use 1× TBE buffer as running buffer as well as to dilute the acrylamide/bisacrylamide solution.

2. Acrylamide/bisacrylamide (19:1) 15 Vol% in 1× TBE, 7 M urea.

3. N, N, N', N'-tetramethylethylenediamine (TEMED) abs.

4. Ammonium persulfate: Prepare 10% (w/v) solution in water and store in the dark at 4 °C.

5. Denaturing loading buffer: 1× TBE, 7 M urea, 50 mM EDTA-Na.

2.14 Dephosphory-lation

1. Product RNA from in vitro transcription purified via PAGE (compare Subheading 3.4): 10 pmol.

2. 1× CIP-Puffer (50 mM potassium acetate, 20 mM Tris-acetate, 10 mM magnesium acetate, 100 µg/mL BSA, pH 7.9 at 25 °C [NEB or single components from Sigma-Aldrich]).

3. CIP (NEB, 1 U/µL).

2.15 5'-Monophos-phorylation

RNA from general in vitro transcription (compare Subheading 3.4) after dephosphorylation (Subheading 3.6) or from chemical synthesis after purification (compare Subheading 3.1 to Subheading 3.3).

1. Non-phosphorylated RNA: 5 pmol.

2. ATP 15 pmol (Thermo Fisher Scientific).

3. Buffer (Tris–HCl [60 mM, pH 8 at 25 °C], 6 mM $MgCl_2$, 10 mM DTE).

4. T4 PNK polynucleotide Kinase (Thermo Fisher Scientific).

2.16 Circularization of Single-Stranded or Partially Single-Stranded RNAs

1. 5'-Monophosphorylated RNA: 2.5 pmol.

2. Buffer (50 mM Tris–HCl, 10 mM $MgCl_2$, 1 mM DTT, pH 7.5 at 25 °C; NEB)

3. ATP (Thermo Fisher Scientific).

4. Enzyme T4 RNA ligase I 10 U (NEB).

2.17   Circularization of Double-Stranded or Partially Double-Stranded RNAs

1. 5′-Monophosphorylated RNA: 4 pmol.
2. Buffer (50 mM Tris–HCl, 2 mM $MgCl_2$, 1 mM DTT, 400 µM ATP, pH 7.5 at 25 °C NEB).
3. ATP 1.5 mM (NEB).
4. Enzyme T4 RNA ligase II (NEB).

2.18   RNA Circularization Control Using RNase R(Hydrolysis of Linear RNA)

1. RNA from ligation mix.
2. $MgCl_2$ 5 mM.
3. Buffer (Tris–HCl 0.2 M (pH 8.0), 1 M KCl, and 1 mM $MgCl_2$).
4. RNase R (10 U, Epicentre).

3   Methods

3.1   Chemical RNA Synthesis and Deprotection

1. Synthesis of RNA is performed on CPG by the phosphoramidite approach using a DNA/RNA synthesizer. The system is kept under argon during the whole procedure. The solutions of phosphoramidites and activator should be kept over molecular sieve (3 Å). The 5-fluorouridine phosphoramidite is incorporated into the growing sequences at the defined position of the substrate.
2. Carry out all synthesis in 1 µmol scale.
3. The reagents and steps in the cycles of the chemical synthesis of RNA according to the phosphoramidite methodology are as follows: detritylation for 36 s, coupling and activation for 6 min, capping for 48 s, and oxidation for 18 s.
4. Carry out all syntheses in the "trityl-off" mode.
5. Place the column containing the solid support with the synthesized RNA in a vial to remove acetonitrile with a table centrifuge.
6. Divide the dry support into two halves and transfer it into two 1.5-mL screw vials.
7. Add 1 mL of a 1:1 (v/v) mixture of 8 M ethanolic methylamine and concentrated NH_3 (30%) to each vial. Tightly close the screw vials. Oligonucleotides up to 20 nt are kept for 40 min at 65 °C; longer oligos are kept for 60 min at 65 °C.
8. Cool down to room temperature and keep conditions for 10 min.
9. Collect the supernatant and wash the support three times with 200 mL of the deprotection solution.
10. Combine all supernatants and dry in a concentrator. Pay attention to the ammonia! At the end of this procedure, only one 1.5-mL vial containing the RNA should result.

11. Flush the vial with the dry RNA pellet with argon and add 800 mL of the desilylation reagent. Be sure that the DMF is really dry. Water will disturb the desilylation reaction and the TBDMS group will not be cleaved off completely.

12. Close the vial with parafilm to airtight and keep conditions at 55 °C for 90 min.

13. Cool down to room temperature, transfer the reaction solution into a 50-mL Falcon tube, and add 200 mL of water to stop the reaction.

14. Add 20 mL of n-butanol; mix it vigorously, and keep the mixture at −20 °C overnight.

15. Centrifuge for 30 min at $7000 \times g$, decant the n-butanol, and dry the pellet in vacuo.

3.2 Purification by Anion-Exchange HPLC (see Note 1)

1. Use the anion-exchange column mentioned in Subheading 2.2 with ÄKTA purifier for the following procedure. The column should be stored in oven at 70 °C all time.

2. Wash the column with two column volumes (cv) buffer A, and 2 cv buffer B (see Subheading 2.6), and then equilibrate with 2 cv buffer A.

3. Make an analytical run with a linear gradient (0%B → 100%B in 6 cv, 2 mL/min) with every RNA. Filter the crude RNA through a 0.2 μm aseptic membrane filter and bring an aliquot up to a volume of 100 mL. Load the column with this sample.

4. Detect the RNA with a UV detector at 254 nm. For preparative scale the linear gradient is changed into a step gradient—depending on the individual separating problem.

5. Load the column with 100 mL of the concentrated crude RNA solution for each HPLC run. Start each run with 1 cv buffer to equilibrate and end with 1 cv buffer B to wash.

6. Collect the fractions containing the desired RNA, combine, desalt by reversed-phase chromatography (*see* Subheading 3.3.3), and dry the oligo in vacuo.

7. For further desalination solve the RNA in 500 mL water and prepare a gel filtration (*see* Subheading 3.3.4).

3.3 Desalination

3.3.1 RNA Precipitation Using Ethanol After Chemical Synthesis

1. Solve the RNA in water and add 20 Vol% 50 mM $MgCl_2$, 10 Vol% 3 M sodium acetate solution (pH 5.3), and 250 Vol% ethanol.

2. Mix the solution and keep it overnight at −20 °C.

3. Centrifuge the precipitate for 20 min at 4000 rpm.

4. Decant the supernatant and wash the RNA pellet with 80% ice-cold ethanol.

5. Dry the pellet for a few minutes in vacuo.

3.3.2 Precipitation of RNA Using Ethanol/ Acetone (see Note 2)

1. Filter the combined elutions with an aseptic filter membrane (0.2 μm), lyophilize, and solve in 2–4 mL water.

2. Add 5 equivalents of ethanol/acetone 1:1 (v/v) to the solution and mix vigorously.

3. Keep the precipitation at −20 °C overnight.

4. Centrifuge the precipitate for 30 min at 6000 rpm.

5. Decant the supernatant and wash the pellet with 500 mL ice-cold ethanol (80%).

6. Dry the pellet for a few minutes in vacuo.

3.3.3 RP Chromatography

1. Wash the Sep-Pak cartridge with 10 mL acetonitrile.

2. Equilibrate the column with 10 mL TBK buffer.

3. Solve the RNA in 0.5–1.0 mL water and load the sample on the column.

4. Wash the column with 2 mL TBK buffer and 20 mL water.

5. Elute the RNA by adding a 3:2 (v/v) mixture of acetonitrile/ water and collect 1 mL fractions (about 10 fractions).

6. Detect the fractions containing the oligonucleotide sample by UV–VIS spectrometry at 254 nm, combine, and dry for a few minutes in vacuo.

3.3.4 Gel Filtration

1. Suspend 1 g Sephadex in 10 mL autoclaved millipore water and let it swell for at least 3 h.

2. Use the swollen gel material to pack a column of 4.0×1.5 cm.

3. Equilibrate the column with 20 mL water.

4. Dissolve the oligonucleotide sample in 500 mL water and load the column.

5. Add slowly 10 mL water to elute the oligonucleotide.

6. Collect 0.5 mL fractions and check for the presence of oligonucleotide by UV–VIS spectrometry at 254 nm.

7. Collect fractions containing RNA.

8. Dry the oligo in vacuo.

3.4 In Vitro Transcription and Product Purification

Carry out all procedures on ice unless otherwise specified.

1. The following protocol describes the in vitro transcription at 50 μL scale; depending on downstream applications scaling up to 2 mL is possible. The given concentrations are final concentrations. This protocol applies if dephosphorylation and rephosphorylation are preferred over in vitro transcription with GMP priming.

2. Mix the necessary volume of water, rNTPs, buffer (1×), and dsDNA template (1 μM) and mix, thoroughly, before adding RiboLock. Mix carefully again, and centrifuge for up to 10 s.

3. Start the reaction by adding T7 RNA polymerase (0.6 U/μL), and mix carefully.

4. Reaction takes place at 37 °C for one up to 3 h. To increase RNA yields, in vitro transcription may also take place overnight.

5. To stop in vitro transcription, hydrolyze the DNA template using DNase I for another 30 min. To increase DNA hydrolysis efficiency, add Mn^{2+} to the reaction mixture and double reaction time.

6. Stop DNA hydrolysis and any residual in vitro transcription by precipitation of the RNA with ice-cold ethanol overnight at −20 °C. Add 250 Vol% of ethanol. For example, if the in vitro transcription was done in a volume of 50 μL, add 125 μL ethanol.

7. Centrifuge the sample for 30–45 min at 40,000 × g at 4 °C. Discard the supernatant and dry the pellet in vacuo. Use a volume of 100–200 μL water for resuspension of the pellet of a single in vitro transcription reaction.

8. Purify the RNA using denaturing polyacrylamide gels. Products of a single in vitro transcription with 50 μL total volume may be purified using a mini gel ($100 \times 80 \times 1.0$ mm³, ca. 15 mL gel solution). Reaction scales up to 2 mL should be purified with $200 \times 150 \times 1.5$ mm³ gels (ca. 80 mL gel solution). Use a 10% aliquot of a single reaction for a mini gel slot. Slots of large gels should not contain more than 75% of a single in vitro transcription reaction with a total volume of 50 μL, although slot may be loaded with higher volumes.

9. Mix gel stock solution with 7 M urea in 1× TBE to obtain 15–20% (v/v) gel solutions. To start the polymerization, add 1% (v/v) of 10% (w/v) ammonium persulfate solution and TEMED (0.1% v/v).

10. To prepare the samples and controls, add 100 Vol% denaturing loading buffer and incubate for 2–5 min at 90 °C.

11. Apply 20 μL of the RNA sample solution to each slot for small gels and 80 μL for large gels, respectively. Use denaturing loading buffer, which additionally contains xylene cyanol and bromophenol blue as marker in one slot.

3.5 In Vitro Transcription with GMP Priming and Product Purification

To obtain 5′-monophosphorylated RNA by enzymatic synthesis use a slightly modified transcription protocol as follows:

1. Identical to Subheading 3.4, **step 1.**

2. Mix the necessary volume of water, CTP, UTP, and ATP (final concentration each: 2 mM), GTP 0.625 mM, GMP 3 mM (*see* **Note 3**), buffer (1×), and dsDNA template (1 μM) and mix, thoroughly, before adding RiboLock. Mix carefully again, and centrifuge for up to 10 s.

3. Identical to Subheading 3.4. **steps 3 to 11**.

**3.6 Dephosphory-
lation of RNA**

When general in vitro transcription (Subheading 3.4) is used, products will have a triphosphate at the 5′-terminus. For ligation, a 5′-monophosphate is required to be covalently linked to a free 3′-hydroxy group. Therefore, the 5′-terminus has to be dephosphorylated prior to 5′-monophosphorylation and ligation.

1. Mix RNA (10 pmol) with buffer (1× = 10 mM Tris–HCl (pH 8.0 at 37 °C), 5 mM $MgCl_2$, 100 mM KCl, 0.02% Triton X-100, and 0.1 mg/mL BSA), 1 U CIP enzyme, and water up to 20 μL.

2. Reaction takes place at 37 °C within 10–15 min. Short reaction time is necessary to avoid alkaline hydrolysis of the RNA due to the alkali buffer.

3. Stop reaction by heating for 5 min at 75 °C and RNA precipitation using ethanol.

**3.7 5′-Phosphory-
lation**

1. Mix RNA (50 pmol) with buffer (1×: 50 mM Tris–HCl [pH 7.6 at 25 °C], 10 mM $MgCl_2$, 5 mM DTT, 0.1 mM spermidine).

2. Add ATP 150 pmol and water up to a volume of 19 μL. You may also use radiolabeled [γ-^{32} or γ-^{33}]-ATP to transfer a radioactive phosphate group to the linear RNA (*see* **Note 4**).

3. Add polynucleotide kinase (10 U).

4. Reaction takes place at 37 °C within 30 min.

5. Stop reaction by heat denaturation at 75 °C for 10 min.

6. When [γ-^{32} or γ-^{33}]-ATP is used, perform gel filtration by Sephadex to get rid of the unlabeled RNA. Use ethanol precipitation to decrease the elution volume.

**3.8 RNA
Circularization with
the Ligation Junction
Positioned in a Single-
Stranded Region**

1. Mix RNA (4 pmol) with buffer 1×, ATP (1 mM) and water up to a volume of 17 μL.

2. Denature at 90 °C for 5 min followed by 50 °C for 5 min.

3. Add 10 U T4 RNA ligase I.

4. Reaction takes place within an hour at 37 °C.

5. Stop reaction by RNA precipitation with ethanol.

**3.9 RNA
Circularization with
the Ligation Junction
Positioned in a
Double-Stranded
Region**

1. Mix RNA (0.36 pmol for a 20 nM reaction or 3.6 pmol for a 200 nM reaction; compare Fig. 3B) with buffer 1×, ATP (1.6 mM) and water up to a volume of 17 μL.

2. Denature at 90 °C for 5 min followed by 50 °C for 5 min.

3. Add 10 U T4 RNA ligase II.

4. Reaction takes place within 3 h at 37 °C.

5. Stop reaction by RNA precipitation with ethanol

3.10 Control of RNA Circularization Using RNase R and PAGE

1. Mix RNA (1 pmol) with buffer 1×, $MgCl_2$ (5 mM), and water up to a volume of 17 μL.

2. Denature at 90 °C for 2 min followed by 50 °C for 2 min.

3. Add RNase R 10 U.

4. Reaction takes place within an hour at 50 °C.

5. Stop reaction by adding 18 μL stop buffer (7 M urea and 50 mM EDTA) .

4 Notes

1. RNA shorter than 20 nt preferentially is purified by HPLC.

2. This method is used for isolation of small RNAs that were purified by PAGE after chemical synthesis.

3. Proportions of GMP:GTP from 5:1 to 40:1 may be used.

4. Ratio of RNA to ATP should be 1:3 or use even more ATP.

References

1. Kulcheski FR, Christoff AP, Margis R (2016) Circular RNAs are miRNA sponges and can be used as a new class of biomarker. J Biotechnol 238:42–51

2. Chen I, Chen CY, Chuang TJ (2015) Biogenesis, identification, and function of exonic circular RNAs. Wiley Interdiscip Rev RNA 6:563–579

3. Zhang Y et al (2013) Circular intronic long noncoding RNAs. Mol Cell 51:792–806

4. Li Z et al (2015) Exon-intron circular RNAs regulate transcription in the nucleus. Nat Struct Mol Biol 22:256–264

5. Danan M, Schwartz S, Edelheit S, Sorek R (2012) Transcriptome-wide discovery of circular RNAs in Archaea. Nucleic Acids Res 40:3131–3142

6. Cortes-Lopez M, Miura P (2016) Emerging functions of circular RNAs. Yale J Biol Med 89:527–537

7. Jeck WR, Sharpless NE (2014) Detecting and characterizing circular RNAs. Nat Biotechnol 32:453–461

8. Qu S et al (2015) Circular RNA: a new star of noncoding RNAs. Cancer Lett 365:141–148

9. Petkovic S, Muller S (2015) RNA circularization strategies in vivo and in vitro. Nucleic Acids Res 43:2454–2465

10. Petkovic S, Muller S (2013) RNA self-processing: formation of cyclic species and concatemers from a small engineered RNA. FEBS Lett 587:2435–2440

11. Harris ME, Christian EL (1999) Use of circular permutation and end modification to position photoaffinity probes for analysis of RNA structure. Methods 18:51–59

12. Petkovic S et al (2015) Sequence-controlled RNA self-processing: computational design, biochemical analysis, and visualization by AFM. RNA 21:1249–1260

Chapter 15

Preparation of Circular RNA In Vitro

Naoko Abe, Ayumi Kodama, and Hiroshi Abe

Abstract

This chapter describes a simple and straightforward way to obtain single-stranded circular RNA sequences in vitro. Linear RNA that is phosphorylated at the 5′ end is first prepared by a chemical or enzymatic method, then circularized using ligase. The function of the prepared circular RNA molecule, such as an ability to induce translation, can then be investigated.

Key words Circular RNA, In vitro transcription, Ligase, Phosphorylation, Polyacrylamide gel electrophoresis

1 Introduction

Recent findings indicate that circular RNAs are abundant in mammalian cells [1]. These endogenous circular RNAs are produced in cells by a splicing reaction, although the detailed mechanism has remained elusive [2]. To understand their function(s), they can be synthesized in vitro and investigated [3]. We found that synthetic circular RNA containing an infinite open reading frame can be translated to produce long polypeptide repeats in mammalian cells in the absence of an internal ribosome entry site element (Fig. 1) [4, 5]. Circular RNA can be prepared both in vitro and in vivo through a splicing reaction of rearranged group I introns in a sequence-dependent manner [6–9]. However, the simplest way to obtain circular RNA in vitro is to prepare a 5′-phosphorylated linear RNA and to circularize it using ligase (Fig. 2) [10]. In this chapter, we first describe how to prepare the precursor linear RNA through chemical or enzymatic synthesis (Figs. 3 and 4). The linear RNA is then circularized using ligase, and the resulting circular RNA is purified for further use by denaturing polyacrylamide gel electrophoresis. The circular RNAs synthesized by this technique would be expected to be several hundred nucleotides in length.

Christoph Dieterich and Argyris Papantonis (eds.), *Circular RNAs: Methods and Protocols*, Methods in Molecular Biology, vol. 1724, https://doi.org/10.1007/978-1-4939-7562-4_15, © Springer Science+Business Media, LLC 2018

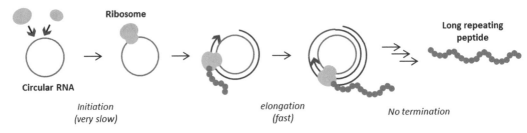

Fig. 1 Schematic of the rolling circle translation on a small circular RNA which contains an infinite open reading frame [4, 5]

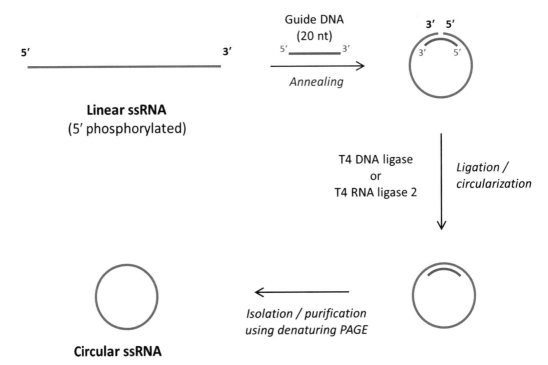

Fig. 2 Schematic of the in vitro preparation of single-stranded (ss) circular RNA using ligase. 5′-phosphorylated linear RNA is joined at its 5′ and 3′ ends onto template DNA

2   Materials

Prepare all solutions using ultrapure water and analytical grade reagents. Prepare and store all reagents at room temperature (unless indicated otherwise). Diligently follow all waste disposal regulations when disposing waste materials.

2.1   Denaturing Polyacrylamide Gel Electrophoresis (PAGE) of RNA

1. Equipment for electrophoresis: A pair of glass plates (20 cm wide × 22 cm high, notched and unnotched), spacers and comb (both 1 mm thickness), clips, electrophoresis apparatus (all from Nihon Eido, Tokyo, Japan) and a power supply (Bio-Rad, Hercules, CA, USA).

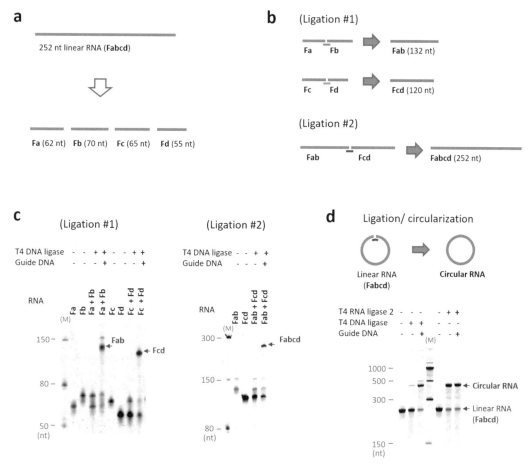

Fig. 3 Schematic of the preparation of 5′-phosphorylated linear RNA based on chemical synthesis (**a–c**) and subsequent circularization of linear RNA (**d**). (**a**) A linear RNA of 252 nt is divided into four RNA fragments (**Fa**, **Fb**, **Fc**, and **Fd**), which are synthesized on an automated DNA/RNA synthesizer using standard phosphoramidite chemistry. All oligomers should be phosphorylated at their 5′ ends on the synthesizer. (**b**) Schematic of the synthesis of linear 252 nt RNA, using RNA oligonucleotides designed in (**a**). First, two oligomers (**Fa** and **Fb**, **Fc** and **Fd**) are joined to produce RNA strands **Fab** and **Fcd**, respectively (Ligation #1). Second, **Fab** and **Fcd** are joined to give fully extended 252 nt RNA **Fabcd** (Ligation #2). (**c**) Denaturing PAGE analysis of the ligation reactions depicted in (**b**). Acrylamide contents in these gels were 8% (*left*) or 6% (*right*). The gels were visualized by SYBR Green II staining. Letter M in the gel denotes the ssRNA size marker. (**d**) Denaturing PAGE (6%) analysis of the circularization reaction of RNA using T4 DNA ligase or T4 RNA ligase 2. The 252 nt linear RNA (**Fabcd** in **b**, **c**) was ligated to circular RNA

2. 0.5 M EDTA (pH 8.0): weigh 93.1 g of ethylenediaminetetraacetic acid disodium salt dihydrate (EDTA·2Na; 0.25 mol) and transfer it to a beaker. Add 0.4 L water to the beaker and stir, then add 10 g of granular NaOH and stir again. Adjust the pH to 8.0 with 5 M NaOH. Make up to 500 mL with water and autoclave.

3. 10× TBE buffer (0.89 M Tris, 0.89 M boric acid, 0.02 M EDTA): weigh 108 g of Tris base (0.89 mol) and 55 g of boric

184   Naoko Abe et al.

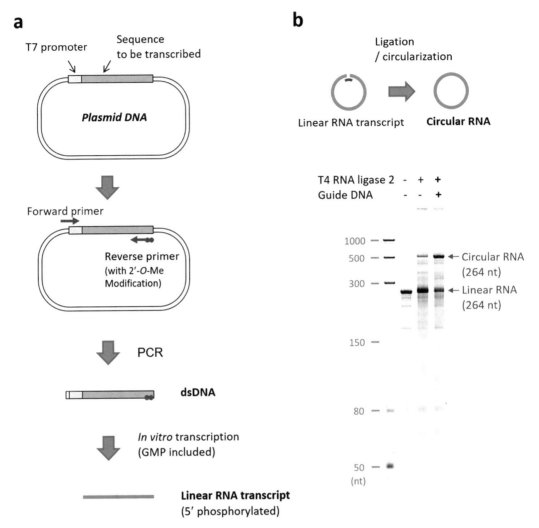

Fig. 4 Schemes of the preparation of 5′-phosphorylated linear RNA by in vitro transcription (**a**), and subsequent circularization of linear RNA (**b**). (**b**) Denaturing PAGE (6%) analysis of the circularization reaction of the 264 nt RNA transcript using T4 RNA ligase 2. The gel was visualized by SYBR Green II staining

acid (0.89 mol) and transfer them to a beaker. Add 0.8 L of water, 40 mL of 0.5 M EDTA (pH 8.0), and stir until the reagents dissolve. Make up to 1 L with water and autoclave. Use 1× TBE as electrophoresis buffer.

4. 2× Formamide gel loading solution [80 (v/v)% formamide, 10 mM EDTA (pH 8.0), 0.02 (w/v)% xylene cyanole FF, 0.02 (w/v)% bromophenol blue]: mix 40 mL of deionized formamide, 1 mL of 0.5 M EDTA (pH 8.0), 10 mg of xylene cyanole FF, and 10 mg of bromophenol blue. Make up to 50 mL with water. Store at 4 °C.

5. 2 × Formamide gel loading solution without dye [80 (v/v)% formamide, 10 mM EDTA (pH 8.0)]: mix 40 mL of deionized formamide and 1 mL of 0.5 M EDTA (pH 8.0). Make up to 50 mL with water. Store at 4 °C. Use this solution when purifying the RNA by PAGE to avoid dye contamination.

6. 40% acrylamide solution (acrylamide: bisacrylamide = 19: 1): weigh 190 g of acrylamide and 10 g of N,N′-methylenebisacrylamide and transfer them to a beaker. Dissolve in water and make up to 500 mL. Store at 4 °C in a light-shielding bottle.

7. 10% denaturing polyacrylamide gel solution [10% acrylamide (acrylamide: bisacrylamide = 19: 1), 7.5 M urea, 25 (v/v)% formamide, 1 × TBE]: mix 10 mL of 40% acrylamide (acrylamide: bisacrylamide = 19: 1), 18.0 g of urea, (0.3 mol) 10 mL of formamide, 4 mL of 10 × TBE. Make up to 40 mL with water (*see* **Note 1**).

8. Ammonium persulfate (APS), 30 (w/v)% solution in water.

9. N,N,N′,N′-Tetramethylethylenediamine (TEMED).

10. Stains-All gel staining solution [0.02 (w/v)% Stains-All in 50% N,N-dimethylformamide].

11. SYBR Green II Nucleic Acid Gel Stain (Lonza, Basel, Switzerland).

12. Low Range ssRNA Ladder (New England Biolabs, Ipswich, MA, USA): size marker of single-stranded RNA for denaturing PAGE analysis.

13. Millex LH filter (pore size, 0.45 μm; disk size, 13 mm; Merck Millipore, Billerica, MA, USA).

14. Amicon Ultra-4 Centrifugal Filters, Ultracel-10 K (Merck Millipore).

15. Amicon Ultra-0.5 Centrifugal Filters, Ultracel-10 K (Merck Millipore).

2.2 Chemical Synthesis of linear 5′-Phosphorylated RNA

1. Standard RNA synthesis reagents: Phosphoramidites [A, U, G, and C-TOM-CE Phosphoramidite (Glen Research, Sterling, VA, USA)] and solid supports [Ac-A-RNA CPG, U-RNA-CPG, Ac-G-RNA CPG and Ac-C-RNA CPG (Glen Research)].

2. Chemical Phosphorylation Reagent (Glen Research).

3. Reagents required for automated DNA/RNA synthesis: Dehydrated acetonitrile, Deblocking Solution, Activator, Cap A, Cap B, and Oxidizing Solution (Glen Research or Wako Pure Chemical (Osaka, Japan)).

4. 33% methylamine in ethanol.

5. 40% aqueous methylamine.

6. Millex LH filter (pore size, 0.45 μm; disk size, 13 mm).

7. Tetrabutylammonium fluoride (TBAF), 1 M solution in tetra-hydrofuran (THF).

8. 1 M Tris–HCl (pH 7.4).

9. NAP-25 column (GE Healthcare, Chicago, IL, USA).

10. 3 M NaOAc (pH 5.2).

11. 20 mg/mL glycogen: add 1 μL of this solution per 1.5/2 mL tube of alcohol-precipitation.

12. Isopropyl alcohol.

13. T4 DNA ligase (Takara Bio, Otsu, Japan).

14. 60 (w/v)% PEG6000: Weigh 0.6 g of PEG6000 and transfer it to a 1.5/2 mL tube with a sealable cap. Add 450 μL of water and heat at 90 °C until it dissolves. The volume will be about 1 mL. Mix thoroughly before use.

15. DNA oligomer(s) of 20-nt as a template for the ligation reaction [11].

2.3   In Vitro Transcription of Linear 5′-Phosphory- Lated RNA

1. Plasmid DNA containing the RNA sequence.

2. A set of PCR primers: substitute two 2′-deoxynucleotides at the 5′-end of the reverse primer with 2′-O-methylated nucleotides (*see* **Note 2**) [12].

3. PrimeSTAR HS DNA Polymerase (Takara Bio).

4. Equipment and reagents for agarose gel electrophoresis (Takara Bio).

5. QIAquick Gel Extraction Kit (Qiagen, Hilden, Germany).

6. MEGAscript T7 Transcription Kit (ThermoFisher Scientific, Waltham, MA, USA) (*see* **Note 3**).

7. 750 mM guanosine 5′-monophosphate (GMP) [10].

2.4   Circularization of 5′-Phosphorylated Linear RNA Using Ligase

1. 5′-phosphorylated linear RNA.

2. DNA oligomer of 20-nt as a template for the ligation reaction.

3. T4 DNA ligase (Takara Bio) or T4 RNA ligase 2 (New England Biolabs).

4. 60 (w/v)% PEG6000.

5. RNase R (Epicentre, Madison, WI, USA).

3   Methods

Carry out all procedures at room temperature unless otherwise specified.

3.1   Preparation of Denaturing Polyacrylamide Gel

First, assemble two glass plates using 1-mm-thick spacers. To 40 mL of 10% denaturing polyacrylamide gel solution, add 120 μL of 30% APS, 40 μL of TEMED, and mix well. Cast the solution between the glass plates immediately. Place a comb between the plates and let the gel polymerize for at least 1 h.

3.2 Analysis and Purification of RNA by Denaturing Polyacrylamide Gelelectrophoresis (PAGE)

1. Add an equal volume of 2 × formamide gel loading solution to the RNA solution.

2. Heat the solution at 90 °C for 3 min. Load the solution onto a 5–10% denaturing polyacrylamide gel.

3. Run the gel at a constant 10–20 W for 1–2 h.

4. Stain the gel for analysis with Stains-All or SYBR Green II dye. If staining with SYBR Green II, visualize the RNA using a gel imaging system and UV excitation.

5. When purifying the RNA, wrap the gel in plastic film, place it on a TLC plate, and detect the RNA using a UV lamp. Mark the band with a marking pen, excise it using a razor blade, and transfer it into a 15 mL tube (or 1.5 mL tube if the gel is smaller than 1 cm^2). Add 4 mL of water to the gel (or 1 mL if the gel is smaller than 1 cm^2) and crush it with a disposable serological pipet (or with a yellow disposable tip). Extract RNA by incubation at room temperature with shaking for 4 h to overnight. After a brief centrifugation, remove the supernatant and store it at 4 °C. Add another 4 mL of water to the crushed gel (or 0.5 mL if the gel is smaller than 1 cm^2), and incubate it for several hours. Remove the supernatant and combine it with the first supernatant. Filter the solution with a Millex LH filter to remove small pieces of gel. Desalt and concentrate the solution using an Amicon Ultra-4 centrifugal device, according to the procedure provided by the manufacturer (or Amicon Ultra-0.5 centrifugal device if the gel is smaller than 1 cm^2). Finally, precipitate the RNA from the concentrated/desalted solution using 3 M NaOAc (pH 5.2) and isopropyl alcohol.

3.3 Chemical Synthesis of linear 5′-Phosphorylated RNA (Fig. 3, See Note 4)

1. Divide the sequence of linear RNA into several, synthesizable lengths. For example, RNA 200 nucleotides in length can be divided into three or four sequences, each of 50–70 nucleotides.

2. Synthesize the RNA lengths on an automated DNA/RNA synthesizer (*see* **Note 5**). RNA oligomers are prepared according to routine phosphoramidite methodology using standard Controlled Pore Glass (CPG) support at the 0.2 or 1 μmol scale. Commercially available 2′-O-triisopropylsilyloxymethyl (TOM) protected amidites [13] are used in our laboratory [5]. For later ligation, phosphorylate RNA 5′ ends on the synthesizer using a commercially available amidite reagent such as Chemical Phosphorylation Reagent [14].

3. Deprotect the oligoribonucleotide [13]. First, add 1 mL of a mixture of 33% methylamine in ethanol/40% methylamine in water (1:1) to the CPG, which was transferred to a 1.5 mL

polypropylene tube with a sealable cap. Incubate this at 35 °C for 6 h or at room temperature overnight. Filter the solution using a Millex LH filter, then dry the filtrate in a vacuum concentrator. Add 1 mL of 1 M TBAF, THF solution to the residue and dissolve it by heating at 50 °C for 10 min with occasional vigorous mixing. Incubate the solution at 35 °C for 6 h or at room temperature overnight. Add 1 mL of 1 M Tris–HCl (pH 7.4) and mix well. Concentrate this in a vacuum concentrator for 30 min until the volume approximates 1 mL. Desalt the solution with a NAP-25 column, using 3 mL of water to elute the RNA. Precipitate the RNA using 3 M NaOAc (pH 5.2) and isopropyl alcohol from the eluate. Dissolve the pellet in water, and determine the RNA concentration by measuring its absorbance at 260 nm.

4. Check the purity of synthesized RNA oligomers by denaturing PAGE (*see* Subheading 3.2).

5. Purify the RNA by preparative denaturing PAGE (*see* Subheading 3.2) (*see* **Note 6**).

6. Ligate synthesized RNA fragments with ligase to a full-length sequence [5]. Design and prepare a guide DNA oligomer of 20-nt which works as a template to join two RNA oligomers. This should be complementary to the 10-nt sequence at the 3′ end of one of the RNA oligomers and to the 10-nt sequence at the 5′ end of the other RNA oligomer. The composition of a typical ligation mixture is: 5 μM RNA fragment_1, 5 μM RNA fragment_2, 7.5 μM guide DNA, 10% PEG6000, 66 mM Tris–HCl (pH 7.6), 6.6 mM MgCl$_2$, 10 mM dithiothreitol (DTT), 0.1 mM ATP, 17.5 U/μL T4 DNA ligase (*see* **Notes 7 and 8**). Mix the two RNA oligomers with the guide DNA oligomer and anneal them by heating at 90 °C for 3 min followed by gradual cooling. Add 60% PEG6000 and T4 DNA ligase and incubate at 37 °C for 4–6 h. Extract the mixture with chloroform to remove PEG6000, which otherwise interferes with denaturing PAGE analysis. Precipitate RNA with 3 M NaOAc (pH 5.2) and isopropyl alcohol in the presence of 20 μg glycogen. Analyze the reaction by 5–10% denaturing PAGE. Identify the slower migrating band that is newly formed by the ligation reaction. Confirm its length by comparing with a commercially available ssRNA ladder marker such as the Low Range ssRNA Ladder. Visualize the RNA by staining the gel with Stains-All or SYBR Green II. Purify the ligated RNA using 10% denaturing PAGE (*see* Subheading 3.2). Repeat the ligation/elongation step until the desired full-length RNA sequence is obtained. Three or four strands of oligoribonucleotides can be ligated simultaneously using two or three guide DNAs, respectively.

3.4 Synthesis of Precursor linear 5′ phosphorylated RNA by In Vitro Transcription (Fig. 4, See Note 4)

1. Construct the transcription template DNA by PCR. First, build a plasmid DNA that can be used as a template in the PCR reaction (Fig. 4a). Include a sequence for the T7 polymerase promoter (5′-TAATACGACTCACTATAG-3′) upstream of the sequence to be transcribed. Ensure that the first base in the transcript is G. Second, carry out a PCR reaction using the plasmid DNA as a template (Fig. 4b). Use an antisense primer modified with 2′-O-methylated nucleotides (see **Note 2**). The composition of a typical PCR reaction mixture is: 0.05 ng/μL plasmid DNA, 1.5 μM of each primer, 0.2 mM dNTPs, 1 × PrimeSTAR Buffer (Mg^{2+} plus), 0.025 U/μL PrimeSTAR HS DNA Polymerase. Run the products on agarose gel electrophoresis. Purify the PCR product using a QIAquick Gel Extraction Kit.

2. Carry out in vitro transcription (Fig. 4b). Add GMP to the reaction mixture to phosphorylate the transcript at its 5′ end [10]. The composition of a typical reaction mixture using the MEGAscript T7 Kit (see **Note 3**) is: 10 ng/μL dsDNA template prepared by PCR, 7.5 mM ATP, 7.5 mM UTP, 7.5 mM CTP, 1.5 mM GTP, 7.5 mM GMP, 1 × Reaction Buffer, 0.1 × Enzyme Mix. Incubate the mixture at 37 °C for 6 h or overnight. Add DNase to the mixture and incubate it at 37 °C for 15 min to degrade the dsDNA template. Desalt/concentrate the mixture using an Amicon Ultra-0.5 10 K centrifugal device. This will eliminate most NTPs and degraded DNA fragments from the mixture. Extract with an equal volume of buffer-saturated phenol/chloroform and then with an equal volume of chloroform. Precipitate the RNA from the aqueous phase using 3 M NaOAc (pH 5.2) and isopropyl alcohol. Dissolve the pellet in water, and determine the RNA concentration by measuring its absorbance at 260 nm. Analyze the transcript by denaturing PAGE. If needed, purify the transcript using preparative denaturing PAGE (see Subheading 3.2).

3.5 Synthesis of Circular RNA by Ligation (Figs. 2, 3d, and 4b)

1. Ligate 5′-phosphorylated linear RNA to form a circle. Design and prepare a guide DNA oligomer of 20-nt which works as a template to join both ends of the linear RNA. The guide DNA oligomer should be complementary to the 10-nt regions at the 5′ and 3′ ends of the RNA. The composition of a typical ligation mixture is: 1 μM 5′-phosphorylated linear RNA, 3 μM guide DNA, 10% PEG6000, 50 mM Tris–HCl, 2 mM MgCl$_2$, 1 mM DTT, 400 μM ATP, pH 7.5, 0.05 U/μL T4 RNA ligase 2 (see **Notes 8** and **9**). Before adding PEG6000 and T4 RNA ligase 2, mix the RNA and guide DNA in the buffer and anneal them by heating at 90 °C for 3 min followed by gradual cooling. Add PEG6000 and T4 RNA ligase 2 and incubate the mixture at 37 °C for 2 h. Extract the mixture with chloroform to remove PEG6000. Precipitate the RNA with 3 M NaOAc

(pH 5.2) and isopropyl alcohol in the presence of 20 μg glycogen. Analyze the reaction by 5%–10% denaturing PAGE (*see* Subheading 3.2, and **Note 10**). Identify the newly formed band in this ligation reaction. In most cases, circularized RNA migrates more slowly than the corresponding linear RNA in denaturing PAGE. Several slower-migrating bands will be formed, although the desired monomeric circular RNA will be the most abundant of these. The others can be attributed to dimeric linear RNA, dimeric circular RNA, and so on. To minimize formation of these undesired products, keep the concentration of linear RNA low in the ligation reaction, specifically below 1 μM [11].

2. Isolate/purify the circular RNA from the mixture described above by preparative denaturing PAGE (*see* **Note 11**) (*see* Subheading 3.2).

3.6   Circularity Check of RNA Using RNase R (Fig. 5, See Note 12)

Treat the possible circular RNA and linear precursor RNA with RNase R, a 3′→5′ exoribonuclease [15], and compare its reactivity by denaturing PAGE analysis. Only linear RNA should be digested. The composition of a typical reaction mixture is: 40 ng/μL RNA, 20 mM Tris–HCl (pH 8.0), 100 mM KCl, 0.1 mM $MgCl_2$, 2 U/μL RNase R. Incubate the mixture at 37 °C for 5–30 min.

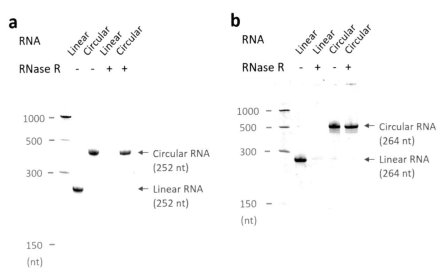

Fig. 5 Circularity check of synthesized circular RNAs by RNase R digestion. PAGE-purified linear/circular RNAs were incubated with RNase R and the reactions were analyzed by denaturing PAGE (6%) analysis. Linear/circular RNAs used in (**a**) or (**b**) correspond to those prepared in Figs. 3 and 4, respectively. The gels were visualized by SYBR Green II staining

4 Notes

1. Change the acrylamide concentration according to the length of RNA analyzed. We changed it from 5 to 10% in these experiments.

2. This modification can reduce undesired non-templated nucleotide addition at the 3′ terminus of RNA upon transcription by T7 RNA polymerase.

3. Use any T7 RNA polymerase available. Set the reaction conditions according to the manufacturer's instructions, but add GMP to the mix. Keep the ratio of [GMP]: [GTP] as 5: 1.

4. 5′-phosphorylated linear RNA can be obtained in two ways, which both have their pros and cons. Chemical synthesis should synthesize circular RNA of a higher purity, but it is more expensive and time-consuming than the enzymatic method (in vitro transcription using T7 RNA polymerase). We recommend opting for the enzymatic method if the circular RNA is longer than 200 nt.

5. Refer to other detailed protocols regarding the synthesis of oligoribonucleotides on an automated synthesizer [16].

6. We use longer gel plates (70 cm long) when purifying chemically synthesized RNA oligomers because longer electrophoresis achieves a higher resolution.

7. Confirm the template-dependency of the ligation reaction to ensure that it proceeds in accordance with the blueprints (the ligation product is not produced by self-dimerization or not inversely connected) (Fig. 3).

8. The addition of PEG6000 is optional. However, its inclusion reduces the amount of enzyme required to complete the reaction.

9. T4 DNA ligase also works in this reaction, although T4 RNA ligase 2 seems to be more efficient. When we used T4 RNA ligase 2 in our laboratory, guide DNA oligomer was not always necessary as a template (*see* Fig. 3d).

10. Optimization of the polyacrylamide content of the gel might be needed to separate circular RNA from its precursor linear RNA.

11. Denaturing PAGE purification can be used to separate/remove guide DNA from circular RNA, which is used as a template in the ligation reaction.

12. Circularity of RNAs can be confirmed by partial digestion of the RNA and following denaturing PAGE analysis of the reaction [5, 11]. An initial cleavage of circular RNA produces a species in the gel that exhibits the same migration as the full-length

cyclization precursor (linear RNA) (refer to Figure 5.2.5 in Reference [13]). Treatment of the possible circular RNA with S1 nuclease or a brief exposure to alkali condition can be used for this purpose.

Acknowledgments

This work was supported by the Ministry of Education, Culture, Sports, Science and Technology of Japan (MEXT).

References

1. Szabo L, Salzman J (2016) Detecting circular RNAs: bioinformatic and experimental challenges. Nat Rev Genet 17:679–692

2. Chen LL (2016) The biogenesis and emerging roles of circular RNAs. Nat Rev Mol Cell Biol 17:205–211

3. Petkovic S, Muller S (2015) RNA circularization strategies in vivo and in vitro. Nucleic Acids Res 43:2454–2465

4. Abe N, Matsumoto K, Nishihara M, Nakano Y, Shibata A, Maruyama H, Shuto S, Matsuda A, Yoshida M, Ito Y, Abe H (2015) Rolling circle translation of circular RNA in living human cells. Sci Rep 5:16435

5. Abe N, Hiroshima M, Maruyama H, Nakashima Y, Nakano Y, Matsuda A, Sako Y, Ito Y, Abe H (2013) Rolling circle amplification in a prokaryotic translation system using small circular RNA. Angew Chem Int Ed 52:7004–7008

6. Ford E, Ares M (1994) Synthesis of circular RNA in bacteria and yeast using RNA cyclase ribozymes derived from a group I intron of phage T4. Proc Natl Acad Sci U S A 91:3117–3121

7. Umekage S, Kikuchi Y (2009) In vitro and in vivo production and purification of circular RNA aptamer. J Biotechnol 139:265–272

8. Perriman R, Ares M (1998) Circular mRNA can direct translation of extremely long repeating-sequence proteins in vivo. RNA 4:1047–1054

9. Perriman R (2002) Circular mRNA encoding for monomeric and polymeric green fluorescent protein. Methods Mol Biol 183:69–85

10. Chen CY, Sarnow P (1995) Initiation of protein-synthesis by the eukaryotic translational apparatus on circular RNAs. Science 268:415–417

11. Diegelman AM, Kool ET (2001) Chemical and enzymatic methods for preparing circular single-stranded DNAs. Curr Protoc Nucleic Acid Chem Chapter 5:Unit 5. 2

12. Kao C, Zheng M, Rudisser S (1999) A simple and efficient method to reduce nontemplated nucleotide addition at the 3′ terminus of RNAs transcribed by T7 RNA polymerase. RNA 5:1268–1272

13. Pitsch S, Weiss PA, Jenny L, Stutz A, Wu XL (2001) Reliable chemical synthesis of oligoribonucleotides (RNA) with 2′-O-(triisopropylsilyl)oxymethyl(2′-O-tom)-protected phosphoramidites. Helv Chim Acta 84:3773–3795

14. Horn T, Urdea MS (1986) A chemical 5′-phosphorylation of oligodeoxyribonucleotides that can be monitored by trityl cation release. Tetrahedron Lett 27:4705–4708

15. Suzuki H, Zuo YH, Wang JH, Zhang MQ, Malhotra A, Mayeda A (2006) Characterization of RNase R-digested cellular RNA source that consists of lariat and circular RNAs from pre-mRNA splicing. Nucleic Acids Res 34:e63

16. Pitsch S, Weiss PA (2002) Chemical synthesis of RNA sequences with 2′-O-[(triisopropylsilyl)oxy]methyl-protected ribonucleoside phosphoramidites. Curr Protoc Nucleic Acid Chem Chapter 3:Unit 3. 8

Chapter 16

Discovering circRNA-microRNA Interactions from CLIP-Seq Data

Xiao-Qin Zhang and Jian-Hua Yang

Abstract

Circular RNAs (circRNAs) represent an abundant group of noncoding RNAs in eukaryotes and are emerging as important regulatory molecules in physiological and pathological processes. However, the precise mechanisms and functions of most of circRNAs remain largely unknown. In this chapter, we describe how to identify circRNA-microRNA interactions from Argonaute (AGO) cross-linking and immunoprecipitation followed by sequencing (CLIP-Seq) and RNA-Seq data using starBase platform and software. We developed three stand-alone computational software, including circSeeker, circAnno, and clipSearch, to identify and annotate circRNAs and their interactions with microRNAs (miRNAs). In addition, we developed interactive Web applications to evaluate circRNA-miRNA interactions identified from CLIP-Seq data and discover the miRNA-sponge circRNAs. starBase platform provides a genome browser to comparatively analyze these interactions at multiple levels. As a means of comprehensively integrating CLIP-Seq and RNA-Seq data, starBase platform is expected to reveal the regulatory networks involving miRNAs and circRNAs. The software and platform are available at http://starbase.sysu.edu.cn/circTools.php.

Key words circRNA, CLIP-Seq, microRNA, Interactome, RNA-Seq, miRNA sponge

1 Introduction

Circular RNAs (circRNAs) are a class of RNA molecules that have a special covalent loop structure without a 5′ cap and 3′ tail [1–3]. CircRNAs are often produced from precursor mRNA (pre-mRNA) back splicing in eukaryotes [1–3]. They are ubiquitously expressed in various tissues and involved in the regulation of gene expression [1–3].

Tens of thousands of circRNAs have been identified by RNA sequencing and bioinformatic approaches [4–11], but determining their functions is an ongoing challenge. To date, only few circRNAs have been experimentally validated with biological functions. The most popular functions of circRNAs are that circRNAs can act as miRNA sponges by sequestering them. The best functionally characterized circRNA is ciRS-7/CDR1-AS [4, 7], which is antisensed to the cerebellar degeneration-related 1 (CDR1) locus (CDR1-AS). The ciRS-7/CDR1-AS is highly expressed in

Christoph Dieterich and Argyris Papantonis (eds.), *Circular RNAs: Methods and Protocols*, Methods in Molecular Biology, vol. 1724, https://doi.org/10.1007/978-1-4939-7562-4_16, © Springer Science+Business Media, LLC 2018

brain and harbors ~70 conserved matches to the miR-7 seed. The knockdown or overexpression of ciRS-7/CDR1-AS leads to marked changes in the levels of known miR-7 targets [4, 7]. A second circRNA proposed to act as a sponge is the testis-specific transcript of the sex-determining gene Sry (circSry), which contains 16 target sites for miR-138 in mouse [4]. In addition to ciRS-7 and cirSry, we also identified several circRNAs containing a considerable number of target sites for miRNAs [12]. However, for the ten thousands of additional and novel circRNAs that have been identified in various species [4–11], which of them will be targeted by miRNAs or act as natural miRNA sponges is currently unclear.

The application of CLIP-Seq methods in Argonaute (AGO) has revealed that various types of linear RNA genes, such as mRNAs and lncRNAs, can be regulated by miRNAs [12–15]. To explore what circRNAs can be targeted by miRNAs, we developed several computational tools to discover circRNAs and their interactions with miRNAs by analyzing the high-throughput AGO CLIP-Seq and RNA-Seq data. We also constructed web interfaces and genome browser to facilitate the analysis of circRNA-miRNA interactions (Fig. 1).

2   Materials

2.1   Hardware

Unix, Windows, or Macintosh workstation with an Internet connection.

2.2   Software

2.2.1   Web Browser

An up-to-date Internet browser, such as Google Chrome (http://www.google.com/chrome), Safari (http://www.apple.com/safari), Internet Explorer (http://www.microsoft.com/windows/internet-explorer/worldwide-sites.aspx), or Firefox (http://www.mozilla.org/firefox), is a basic need.

2.2.2   circSeeker Software

circSeeker is a software for discovering circRNAs from long RNA-Seq or long CLIP-Seq sequences [12, 16]. It has been used to identify circRNAs from long RNA-Seq generated from various tissues/cell lines [12, 16].

2.2.3   circAnno Tool

circAnno is a software for annotating the exon boundaries and containing the exons from known gene annotation. It has been used to annotate the novel circRNAs deposited in starBase and deepBase platforms.

2.2.4   clipSearch Software

clipSearch is a software for identifying the interactions between circRNAs and miRNAs from CLIP-Seq datasets by searching the seed matches in AGO-binding sites. It has been used to identify circRNA-miRNA interactions in starBase platform [12, 17].

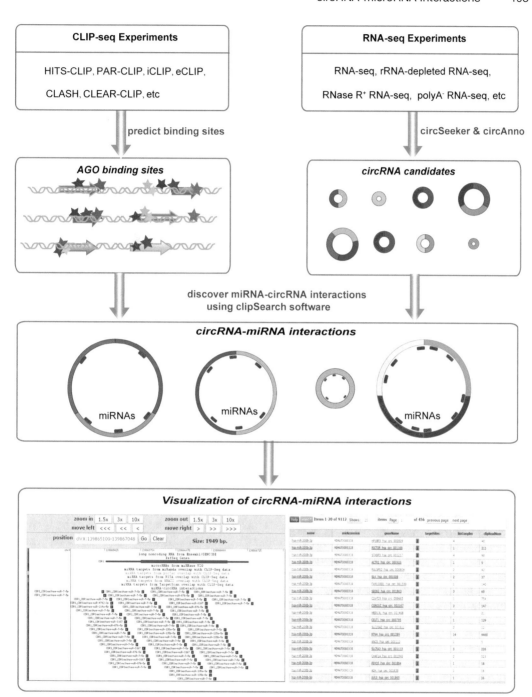

Fig. 1 Basic framework for identifying circRNA-miRNA interactions from CLIP-Seq and RNA-Seq data. Stand-alone software for identifying the circRNAs and their interactions with miRNAs are provided in starBase platform. All results generated by this framework are displayed in the visual browser and web page

2.3 Downloading the Software

The circSeeker, circAnno, and clipSearch are freely available from the following URL: http://starbase.sysu.edu.cn/circTools.php. Choose the appropriate platform for a binary distribution or "src" for the source distribution.

2.4 Installing the Software

2.4.1 Installing a Binary Distribution

After downloading the binary distribution that is appropriate for the specific platform, unpack it, and copy the binary to the desired directories.

2.4.2 Compiling and Installing Software Under Unix

This section explains the compilation and installation of the circSeeker source distribution in a Unix environment, such as Solaris, Linux, Windows Cygwin, or Mac OS X. Similar procedures can be applied in other tools: (1) Unzip and extract the file: tar–xvzf circSeeker-0.1.tar.gz. This should create a directory named circSeeker-0.1, which contains the whole distribution. (2) Compile the program: make. The binary file has been copied to the bin directory (*see* **Note 1**).

2.5 Data Sources

Primary data sources of the CLIP-Seq data and predicted circRNA-miRNA interactions have been deposited in our starBase platform [12, 17]. User can download these data in starBase downloading center (http://starbase.sysu.edu.cn/download.php, *see* also **Note 2**).

3 Methods

The methods presented in this chapter describe how to discover circRNA-miRNA interactions from AGO CLIP-Seq and RNA-Seq data, and how to use starBase web interface to retrieve the interactions and run a comparative analysis of these data using the deepView genome browser (Fig. 1).

3.1 Discovering circRNAs from RNA-Seq Sequencing Data

To study what circRNAs can be targeted by the miRNAs, we first identified circRNAs from long RNA-Seq datasets. In this section, we summarize the features and workflow used to identify circRNAs from long RNA-Seq data by our circSeeker software. In brief, the circSeeker searches the junction read that is aligned to two different locations in the same chromosome and same strand. For each junction read, only the sum length of left segment and right segment that is greater than or equal to the total length of read was kept. circSeeker further adjusts the length of two segments from junction read to determine the precise positions of downstream donor and upstream acceptor splice sites, respectively (Fig. 2a). The following steps describe how to use the circSeeker to discover circRNAs in the human genome (this workflow is also applicable for other species) from high-throughput RNA-Seq data.

1. Next-generation sequencing data processing. Remove 3′ adapters or barcodes from raw sequencing data with FASTQ format (*see* **Note 3**). User can remove adapters and barcodes of raw sequencing data using the FASTX-Toolkit or cutadapt software [18]. To remove the low-quality reads, we set a read quality for each dataset, retaining only those reads with a quality score above 20 in 80% of their nucleotides. For paired-end sequencing data, read1 and read2 files should be merged into one.

2. Collapsing the reads: To reduce the run time for aligning the reads and discovering circRNAs, the same reads are collapsed into unique reads (*see* **Note 4**). Reads can be collapsed using FASTX-Toolkit tool. This is an optional step for circSeeker software.

3. Genome sequences and faidx file preparation: User can download the genome from public genome centers, such as UCSC Bioinformatics or ENSEMBL websites. User can use the samtools faidx command to generate faidx file of genome [19]. The faidx file (*see* **Note 5**) will help the program to fast fetch the subsequence of genome.

4. Mapping processed reads to reference genome and keeping the unmapped reads: User may select various ultrafast aligners to map the reads to reference genomes. Recent studies have found that there are many mismatches and indels in long RNA-Seq data [20]. Thus, it will be better to select an aligner that allows mismatches and indels, such as bowtie2 [21], STAR [22], and BWA [23]. In this chapter, we used bowtie2 as an example to map reads to human genome. Before aligning the reads to genome, users should build the index file of genome with bowtie2-build program [21]. The reads are aligned to human genome (version hg19) using bowtie 2.0 (parameters: -D 200 -R 3 -N 0 -L 20 -i S,1,0.5 –score-min = C,-16,0). The aligned reads are discarded and the remaining unmapped RNA-Seq reads are used to identify circRNAs.

5. Mapping unmapped reads to genome with local model: The unmapped reads were aligned again using bowtie2 with the parameters (−−no-unal –local –reorder -k 20 -D 200 -R 3 -N 0 -L 20 -i S,1,0.5) and then converted alignment SAM format into the BAM format (*see* **Note 6**) sorted by name using samtools program [19].

6. Predicting circRNAs from the alignments of unmapped reads: Start circSeeker with the following options: circSeeker –o circRNA_candidates.txt genome.fa genome.fai unmapped. reads.bam. Users can set the options to filter the candidates. For example, the option -d 300,000 tells circSeeker to output the circRNAs with less than 300,000 spanning distance only (*see* also **Note 1**). You can set more options for circSeeker (Fig. 2b). After a short time (*see* **Note 7**), the circSeeker

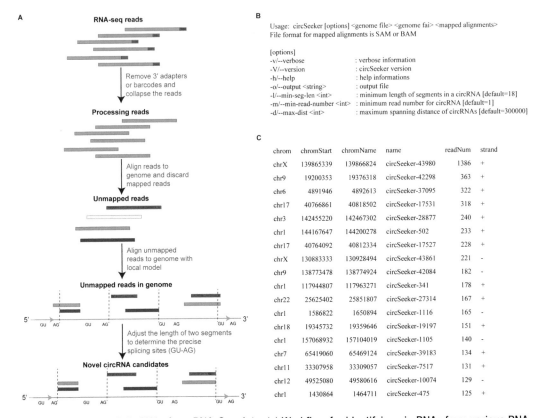

Fig. 2 Identification of circRNAs from RNA-Seq data. (**a**) Workflow for identifying circRNAs from various RNA-Seq data. The workflow is divided into several main stages, including data processing, data mapping, and splicing-site determination. (**b**) The usage of circSeeker software. The various options are displayed. (**c**) The output results of circSeeker. Only six columns are shown

program will output the results (Fig. 2c). The output includes chromosome, genome location, and number of reads spanning the junctions.

3.2 Annotating circRNAs Using circAnno Software

The computational tools for the identification of circRNAs only output the start and end positions of circRNAs and could not determine how many exons the circRNAs contain. In this section, we summarize the features and workflow used to annotate the circRNAs (Fig. 3a).

1. Preparing the gene annotations: The annotation file with BED12 format (*see* **Note 8**) can be fetched for circAnno in the UCSC Genome Browser website by the following steps: Open a UCSC Table Browser (http://genome.ucsc.edu/cgi-bin/hgTables) and perform a species selection by specifying clade, genome, and assembly. Select "Genes and Gene Predictions" group, "GENCODE Gene" track, and a relevant "Comprehensive" table. In the "output format" panel of UCSC table, select

"BED-browser extensible data". Finally, click "get output" button; a BED12 file will be returned as an output.

2. Annotating novel circRNAs using the known gene annotation. Run circAnno with the following options: circAnno -m -o circAnno_candidates.txt genes.bed12 circRNAs.bed6. Similarly, the user can set the option to output different results. For example, the option -m tells circAnno to only output the circRNAs that map the precise exon boundaries of known genes. You can use option -h to view more options for circAnno (Fig. 3b). After a very short time (*see* also **Note 7**), the program will return the results.

3. Displaying the annotated circRNAs in the genome browser. Given that circAnno outputs the BED12 file, user can upload the file in UCSC Genome Browser and display the circRNAs in genome browser with the following steps: Open the "Add Custom Tracks" page (http://genome.ucsc.edu/cgi-bin/hgCustom) and perform a species selection as described in Subheading 3.2, **step 1**. Click "upload" button to select the annotated circRNA file. And then click the "Submit" button to upload the file to genome browser. Finally, the custom-tracked annotated circRNAs will be displayed in the genome browser. An example is shown in Fig. 3c.

3.3 Predicting
AGO-Binding Sites
from CLIP-Seq Data

High-throughput CLIP-Seq method provides a powerful way to identify the AGO-binding sites. In this section, we summarize the features and workflow used to identify Argonaute-binding sites from CLIP-Seq data. The general computational workflow summary from a series of recent publications [24–27] is as follows (Fig. 4a):

1. CLIP-Seq data processing: As described in Subheadings 3.1, **step 1**, remove 5′ and 3′ adapters or barcodes from raw deep sequencing data. The same reads were collapsed into unique reads.

2. Mapping processed CLIP-Seq reads to reference genome: According to different CLIP-Seq experimental methods, the user may select different ultrafast aligners. As frequently inductions of mutations and indels in UV cross-link experiments, it will be better to select aligners that allow mismatches and indels, such as bowtie2 [21] and BWA [23].

3. Discovering the AGO-binding sites: (1) For PAR-CLIP, the cross-link sites often include transitions from thymidine to cytidine (T → C) in the resulting cDNA; the clusters therefore must include one or more (T → C) mutations [26]. In starBase, the AGO PAR-CLIP was analyzed using PARalyzer software (v1.1) [23]. (2) For CLIP-Seq, several methods have been proposed to evaluate the statistical significance of AGO-binding peaks [24–27]. For example, Yeo et al. identified bind-

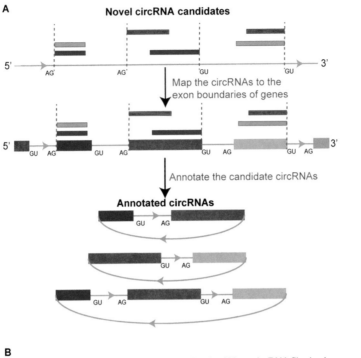

B

Usage: circAnno [options] <annotation file, bed12> <circRNA file, bed>
File format for bed is bed6 or bed12

[options]
-v/--verbose   : verbose information
-V/--version   : circAnno version
-h/--help   : help informations
-m/--match   : only output the circRNAs with matched splice sites[default,output all]
-i/--min-len   : minimum length of circRNA transcript[default=50]
-x/--max-len   : maximum length of circRNA transcript[default=300000]
-o/--output <string> : output file

C

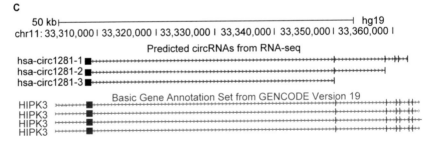

Fig. 3 Annotation of circRNAs using circAnno software. (**a**) Workflow for annotating circRNAs that are identified by circSeeker. The workflow is divided into several main steps, including mapping the locations to exon boundaries, and determining the exons of circRNAs. (**b**) The usage of circAnno software. The various options are displayed. (**c**) The output results of circAnno are displayed in the UCSC Genome Browser

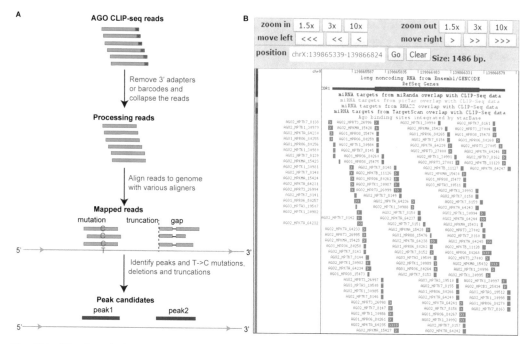

Fig. 4 Identification of AGO-binding peaks from CLIP-Seq data. (**a**) Workflow for identifying Argonaute-binding sites from CLIP-Seq data. The workflow is divided into several main stages, including data processing, data mapping, data filter, and identification of mutations, deletions, truncations, and binding sites from CLIP-Seq data. (**b**) The CLIP-Seq peaks are shown in the starBase Genome Browser

ing sites using Poisson distribution model and filtered the candidates using false discovery rate (FDR) [25]. Recently, several studies used the information of mutations, truncations, and deletions to map the AGO-binding sites at single-nucleotide resolution [27]. In starBase, the AGO CLIP-identified binding site clusters/peaks are integrated and used directly. All AGO CLIP-Seq peaks are stored in MYSQL database and displayed in our starBase Genome Browser (Fig. 4b).

3.4 Identifying the circRNA-miRNA Interactions Using clipSearch Software

To identify target sites of miRNA from CLIP-Seq data, the clipSearch program was developed to search for 6–8mers (8-mer, 7-mer-m8, and 7-mer-A1) in CLIP-Seq peaks [17]. This tool starts by scanning peak clusters for potential miRNA targets (6–8mers), folding the miRNA-target duplex and calculating the minimum free energy (MFE), scoring the alignments generated by Needleman-Wunsch algorithm, and then outputting the detailed information (Fig. 5a). In this section, we introduce how to use clipSearch program to predict target sites of miRNAs from CLIP-Seq data.

1. Predicting miRNA target sites in peaks: Start clipSearch with the following options: clipSearch –o miRNA_targets.txt genome.fa genome.fai miRNA.fa AGO_peaks.bed6. The user

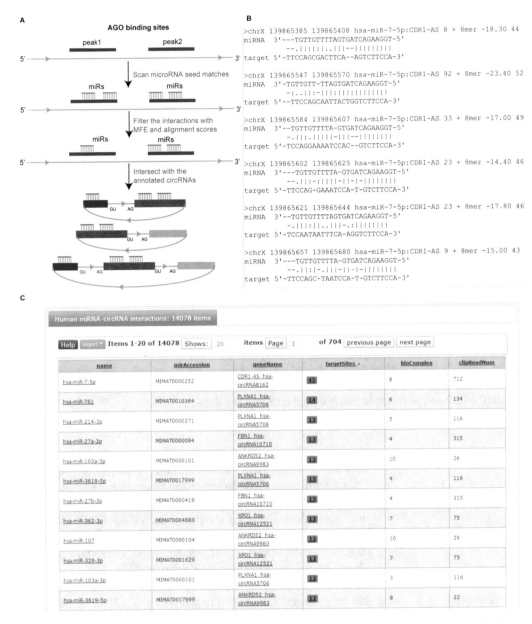

Fig. 5 Prediction of circRNA-miRNA interactions using clipSearch software. (**a**) Workflow for predicting the interactions between miRNAs and circRNAs from AGO-binding peaks. (**b**) The output results of clipSearch software. The output includes genomic information, aligned score, MFE, and alignments between miRNAs and circRNAs. (**c**) A screenshot of circRNA-miRNA interaction page

can employ multiple options to limit the output results. For example, the option -m −10.0 tells clipSearch to just output the minimum free energy (MFE) with less than −10.0 kcal/mol. You can use option -h or open the README file to view and then set more options for clipSearch. After a short time (*see* also **Note** 7), the program will return the detailed results (Fig. 5b).

2. Associating the miRNA target sites with circRNAs: User can use bedtools (http://bedtools.readthedocs.io/en/latest/) to identify which target sites are overlapping with and located within exons of circRNAs.

3. Conservation of circRNA–miRNA interactions: The target sites predicted by clipSearch in BED format can be examined for their conservation in the UCSC Genome Browser website following the next steps: As described in Subheading 3.2, **step 1**, open a UCSC Table Browser and select the species. And then select "Comparative Genomics" group and a conservation table (e.g., phyloP scores). In the "region" panel of UCSC Table Browser, select "define region" to upload the BED file of miRNA target sites. Finally, click the "summary/statistics" button; a summary page with each target site conservation is returned as an output.

3.5 Browsing circRNA-miRNA Interactions Predicted by ClipSearch

We constructed the first platform that provided a comprehensive collection of >10,000 CLIP-Seq that experimentally supported circRNA-miRNA interactions (*see* **Note 9**). The following steps describe how to use the starBase website to evaluate the circRNA-miRNA interactions overlapping with CLIP-Seq data.

1. Click "miRNA-lncRNA->miRNA-circRNA interactions" to open the circRNA-miRNA interaction page.

2. Select the clade, genome, and assembly of interest. For example, choose the "mammal->human->hg19".

3. If you want to search what circRNAs are targeted by the miRNA of interest, you can select the specific miRNA (e.g., hsa-mir-7-5p). If you want to search what miRNAs target the circRNA of interest, you can enter the circRNA name (e.g., CDR1-AS).

4. Some CLIP-Seq peaks with small read numbers may simply represent experimental or biological noises, so we provide an option to allow users to further filter these target sites by limiting the number of supporting CLIP-Seq experiments.

5. Finally, you can click "Search" to see a list of circRNA-miRNA interactions in the human genome. The miRNA name and accession, official circRNA gene name, number of experiments, and number of target sites and CLIP-Seq reads are indicated in a table (Fig. 5c). The user can click on the title of the table to sort circRNA-miRNA interactions according to various features, such as the number of reads, miRNA names, bioComplex (also called the number of experiments), gene names, and target sites.

6. Click on the nonzero target sites within the table to launch a detailed page providing further information on that circRNA-miRNA interaction. The detailed information for an interaction includes (1) a description of the target gene, CLIP-Seq cluster overlapping with target site, number of CLIP-Seq, alignScore, MFE, and alignment between miRNA and circRNA. (2) Click the target location to view the genomic context of the target site in our starBase genome browser. (3) Click the CLIP-Seq peak; user can view the peak location, CLIP type, study, cell line, treatment, and accession number. (4) The "study" section enables the retrieval of the primary articles yielded from the CLIP-Seq sequencing data.

7. Identifying the circRNAs as "super-sponges" of miRNAs: It has been reported that ciRS-7/CDR1-AS circRNA acts as a super miR-7 sponge that contains multiple target sites from the same miRNA; user can test whether the other circRNAs hosted in our database can act as super miRNA sponges. User can sort the circRNA-miRNA web page by the target sites to discover how many target sites are in one circRNA. We can recapitulate the known CDR1as circRNA as a miR-7 super-sponge using the miRNA-circRNA interaction web page (Fig. 5c). In addition, our platform also identified more than 20 circRNAs that harbored >10 target sites of the same miRNA.

3.6 Comparative Analysis of circRNA-miRNA Interactions Using starBase Genome Browser

To facilitate the visualization of AGO CLIP-Seq datasets and exploration of circRNA-miRNA interactions, we provided starBase Genome Browser that was written using a GD graphics library for PHP. In the query page of the browser, users can input one interested genomic region or gene name in the "search term" and select corresponding genome assembly to gain an integrated view of various genomic features. A sample screenshot for the output of the starBase Genome Browser can be found at URL http://starbase.sysu.edu.cn/browser.php. User can zoom into a region of interest and proceed to a detailed view of track item within the browser by clicking it. Moreover, the "zoom out" or "zoom in" button can be used to extend or shrink the width of the displayed coordinate range.

To explore the miRNA target sites on a particular circRNA, users can type its gene symbol in the position textbox and then click the "GO" button to update the display image and to determine what target sites are located within the circRNA. In addition, user can click a check box and click "Refresh Tracks" button to display AGO binding track of interest, and then determine whether this circRNA can also be bound by AGO proteins.

4   Notes

1. Compile the program. The source codes (circSeeker, circAnno, and clipSearch) were written by C/C++ programming language and can easily be compiled with the GNU C++ compiler gcc in version 4.4.7. 3. The circSeeker, circAnno, and clipSearch distributions contain README documents to explain all parameters and how to run the programs. By following the installation procedure of Subheading 2.4, the README files will be extracted in the program directory.

2. The sequence and annotation data is in UCSC BED. The circRNA-miRNA interaction file in the BED format includes chromosome, start position, end position, circRNA name, score, and strand direction. It should be noted that all start coordinates are 0 based in the starBase database. Users can upload these files to the UCSC Genome Browser and display them in the UCSC Genome Browser.

3. The format of raw read is FASTQ. Each read entry consists of four lines. Line 1 begins with a "@" character and is followed by a sequence identifier. Line 2 is the raw sequence letters. Line 3 begins with a "+" character and is often followed by the same sequence identifier. Line 4 encodes the quality values for the sequence in Line 2, and must contain the same number of symbols as letters in the sequence.

4. The format of collapsed read is FASTA format. It begins with the symbol ">" followed by the read's identifier and then the read itself. For example, in the format of ">10–15 GCACCTGTGTCA", "10" represents a FASTX-Toolkit unique ID for unique reads, and "15" indicates that this read [10] has been detected 15 times in the RNA sequencing dataset. Both of them are linked by a hyphen.

5. Fai index file: The fai index file is a text file consisting of lines each with five TAB-delimited columns. Please see detailed information at URL http://www.htslib.org/doc/faidx.html.

6. SAM and BAM format: SAM represents Sequence Alignment/Map format. It is a TAB-delimited text format consisting of a header section, which is optional, and an alignment section. BAM is the binary format of SAM file. Please visit the following website (http://genome.sph.umich.edu/wiki/SAM) to see the detailed information.

7. Approximate runtime (1) circSeeker: After mapping the reads to genome, circSeeker will be very fast. Searching BAM file with 60 Gb, circSeeker takes only 30 min. (2) circAnno: Annotating >100,000 circRNAs, circAnno takes only 2 min. (3) clipSearch: Searching target sites of 277 conserved miR-

NAs in ~1,000,000 AGO-binding peaks, clipSearch takes 50 min.

8. BED12 format: BED (Browser-Extensible Data) format provides an efficient way to define the data lines, and is considered as a widely accepted input format for many tools and databases. The detailed information is as follows: URL: http://genome.ucsc.edu/FAQ/FAQformat.html#format1.

9. In starBase, all circRNA-miRNA interactions are stored in related tables of MySQL database. A specific naming convention has been used for each circRNA. Take human as an example: circRNAs are designated with accession (e.g., hsa-circRNA108-3): the "hsa" stands for "Homo sapiens", "circRNA108" stands for "circRNA family", and the following "3" stands for "isoform number".

Acknowledgments

This research is supported by the National Natural Science Foundation of China (No. 31370791, 91440110); Funds from Guangdong Province (No. S2012010010510, S2013010012457); the project of Science and Technology New Star in ZhuJiang Guangzhou city (No. 2012J2200025); Fundamental Research Funds for the Central Universities (No. 2011330003161070, 14lgjc18); China Postdoctoral Science Foundation (No. 200902348); and seeding project fund at School of Medicine, South China University of Technology (yxy2016005). This research is supported in part by the Guangdong Province Key Laboratory of Computational Science and the Guangdong Province Computational Science Innovative Research Team.

References

1. Jeck WR, Sharpless NE (2014) Detecting and characterizing circular RNAs. Nat Biotechnol 32:453–461

2. Chen LL (2016) The biogenesis and emerging roles of circular RNAs. Nat Rev Mol Cell Biol 17:205–211

3. Szabo L, Salzman J (2016) Detecting circular RNAs: bioinformatic and experimental challenges. Nat Rev Genet 17:679–692

4. Hansen TB, Jensen TI, Clausen BH, Bramsen JB, Finsen B, Damgaard CK, Kjems J (2013) Natural RNA circles function as efficient microRNA sponges. Nature 495:384–388

5. Zhang XO, Wang HB, Zhang Y, Lu X, Chen LL, Yang L (2014) Complementary sequence-mediated exon circularization. Cell 159:134–147

6. Liang D, Wilusz JE (2014) Short intronic repeat sequences facilitate circular RNA production. Genes Dev 28:2233–2247

7. Memczak S, Jens M, Elefsinioti A, Torti F, Krueger J, Rybak A, Maier L, Mackowiak SD, Gregersen LH, Munschauer M, Loewer A, Ziebold U, Landthaler M, Kocks C, le Noble F, Rajewsky N (2013) Circular RNAs are a large class of animal RNAs with regulatory potency. Nature 495:333–338

8. Jeck WR, Sorrentino JA, Wang K, Slevin MK, Burd CE, Liu J, Marzluff WF, Sharpless NE (2013) Circular RNAs are abundant, con-

served, and associated with ALU repeats. RNA 19:141–157

9. You X, Vlatkovic I, Babic A, Will T, Epstein I, Tushev G, Akbalik G, Wang M, Glock C, Quedenau C, Wang X, Hou J, Liu H, Sun W, Sambandan S, Chen T, Schuman EM, Chen W (2015) Neural circular RNAs are derived from synaptic genes and regulated by development and plasticity. Nat Neurosci 18:603–610

10. Li Z, Huang C, Bao C, Chen L, Lin M, Wang X, Zhong G, Yu B, Hu W, Dai L, Zhu P, Chang Z, Wu Q, Zhao Y, Jia Y, Xu P, Liu H, Shan G (2015) Exon-intron circular RNAs regulate transcription in the nucleus. Nat Struct Mol Biol 22:256–264

11. Hentze MW, Preiss T (2013) Circular RNAs: splicing's enigma variations. EMBO J 32: 923–925

12. Li JH, Liu S, Zhou H, Qu LH, Yang JH (2014) starBase v2.0: decoding miRNA-ceRNA, miRNA-ncRNA and protein-RNA interaction networks from large-scale CLIP-Seq data. Nucleic Acids Res 42:D92–D97

13. Konig J, Zarnack K, Luscombe NM, Ule J (2011) Protein-RNA interactions: new genomic technologies and perspectives. Nat Rev Genet 13:77–83

14. Fu XD, Ares M Jr (2014) Context-dependent control of alternative splicing by RNA-binding proteins. Nat Rev Genet 15:689–701

15. Darnell RB (2010) HITS-CLIP: panoramic views of protein-RNA regulation in living cells. WIREs RNA 1:266–286

16. Zheng LL, Li JH, Wu J, Sun WJ, Liu S, Wang ZL, Zhou H, Yang JH, Qu LH (2016) deep-Base v2.0: identification, expression, evolution and function of small RNAs, LncRNAs and circular RNAs from deep-sequencing data. Nucleic Acids Res 44:D196–D202

17. Yang JH, Li JH, Shao P, Zhou H, Chen YQ, Qu LH (2011) starBase: a database for exploring microRNA-mRNA interaction maps from Argonaute CLIP-Seq and Degradome-Seq data. Nucleic Acids Res 39:D202–D209

18. Martin M (2011) Cutadapt removes adapter sequences from high-throughput sequencing reads. EMBnet. J 17(1):10

19. Li H, Handsaker B, Wysoker A, Fennell T, Ruan J, Homer N, Marth G, Abecasis G, Durbin R (2009) The sequence alignment/map format and SAMtools. Bioinformatics 25:2078–2079

20. Wang Z, Gerstein M, Snyder M (2009) RNA-Seq: a revolutionary tool for transcriptomics. Nat Rev Genet 10:57–63

21. Langmead B, Salzberg SL (2012) Fast gapped-read alignment with Bowtie 2. Nat Methods 9:357–359

22. Dobin A, Davis CA, Schlesinger F, Drenkow J, Zaleski C, Jha S, Batut P, Chaisson M, Gingeras TR (2013) STAR: ultrafast universal RNA-seq aligner. Bioinformatics 29:15–21

23. Li H, Durbin R (2009) Fast and accurate short read alignment with burrows-wheeler transform. Bioinformatics 25:1754–1760

24. Chi SW, Zang JB, Mele A, Darnell RB (2009) Argonaute HITS-CLIP decodes microRNA-mRNA interaction maps. Nature 460: 479–486

25. Zisoulis DG, Lovci MT, Wilbert ML, Hutt KR, Liang TY, Pasquinelli AE, Yeo GW (2010) Comprehensive discovery of endogenous Argonaute binding sites in Caenorhabditis elegans. Nat Struct Mol Biol 17:173–179

26. Hafner M, Landthaler M, Burger L, Khorshid M, Hausser J, Berninger P, Rothballer A, Ascano M Jr, Jungkamp AC, Munschauer M, Ulrich A, Wardle GS, Dewell S, Zavolan M, Tuschl T (2010) Transcriptome-wide identification of RNA-binding protein and microRNA target sites by PAR-CLIP. Cell 141: 129–141

27. Zhang C, Darnell RB (2011) Mapping in vivo protein-RNA interactions at single-nucleotide resolution from HITS-CLIP data. Nat Biotechnol 29:607–614

Chapter 17

Identification of circRNAs for miRNA Targets by Argonaute2 RNA Immunoprecipitation and Luciferase Screening Assays

Yan Li, Bing Chen, and Shenglin Huang

Abstract

Circular RNAs from back-spliced exons (circRNAs) represent a novel class of widespread and endogenous RNAs in eukaryotes. circRNAs may bind to microRNAs (miRNAs) and inhibit the activity of miRNAs. Alternatively, miRNAs could also directly target circRNAs and regulate the expression of circRNAs. Here we describe the Argonaute2 (AGO2) RNA immunoprecipitation (RIP) and luciferase screening assays to identify the interaction between circRNAs and miRNAs. The AGO2 RIP assay evaluates the potential of the interaction between circRNAs and miRNAs. The luciferase screening assay investigates the targeting miRNAs and the detail binding sites for a specific circRNA.

Key words Circular RNA, microRNA, RNA immunoprecipitation, Luciferase screening assay

1 Introduction

Circular RNAs (circRNAs) are covalently closed and single-stranded transcripts that are produced from precursor mRNA back splicing in eukaryotes. The recent application of high-throughput RNA sequencing and bioinformatics approach has revealed a large number of circRNAs in different species [1–4]. Although they are generally expressed at low levels, emerging evidence has demonstrated that certain circRNAs are linked to physiological development and various diseases, such as neurological dystrophy [3], cardiovascular diseases [5–7], and cancer [8–10]. The general mechanisms of circRNAs remain elusive. However, recent findings have indicated that circRNAs may interact with RNA or proteins and serve as transcription or splicing regulators [11, 12]. Particularly, circRNAs have been found to interact with microRNA (miRNA) and function as miRNA sponges. The typical example is CDR1as circRNA, which harbors about 60 conserved binding sites for miR-7 [13, 14]. The testis-specific circRNA, sex-determining

Christoph Dieterich and Argyris Papantonis (eds.), *Circular RNAs: Methods and Protocols*, Methods in Molecular Biology, vol. 1724, https://doi.org/10.1007/978-1-4939-7562-4_17, © Springer Science+Business Media, LLC 2018

region Y (circSRY), contains 16 target sites for miR-138 in mice [13]. However, only a few of such circular RNAs contain multiple binding sites to trap a particular miRNA. Recent publications have suggested that circRNAs do not necessarily function as miRNA sponges in human and mouse cells [2–4, 15]. Nevertheless, circular RNAs in Drosophila reportedly contain conserved miRNA sites. Notably, one circRNA may be associated with a variety of miRNAs, as shown with circHIPK3 and circ-Foxo3 [8, 16], which can bind to multiple miRNAs. Such an interaction would be more common for circRNAs that are associated with miRNAs. Thus, circRNA may, but not generally, function as sponge for miRNA. Alternatively, miRNAs could also directly target circRNAs and regulate the expression of circRNAs. For example, miR-671 can bind to CDR1as and trigger the destruction of CDR1as [17]. The circRNA-miRNA interaction is mediated by the RNA-induced silencing complex (RISC) containing Argonaute2 (AGO2) and many associated proteins. The detection of circRNA from AGO2 RNA immunoprecipitation (RIP) assay may examine whether the circRNA candidate could bind to miRNAs. In this chapter, we describe the AGO2 RIP and luciferase screening assays to identify the interaction between circRNAs and miRNAs. The schematic illustration of the methodology is shown in Figs. 1 and 2.

2   Materials

2.1   AGO2 RNA Immunoprecipitation

1. 1×Phosphate-buffered saline (PBS): 1.37 mM NaCl, 2.6 mM KCl, 10 mM Na_2HPO_4, 1.8 mM KH_2PO_4. Adjust the pH to 7.4 with HCl.

2. RIP lysis buffer: 50 mM Tris–HCl PH 7.4, 150 mM NaCl, 1 mM EDTA, 0.5% NP-40, 5% glycerine.

3. Recombinant RNase Inhibitor (TakaRa).

4. 1× Protein SDS-PAGE loading buffer.

5. Protein-G-coated beads (Life Technologies).

6. Anti-Argonaute-2 (Abcam ab57113).

7. TRIzol (Life Technologies, Carlsbad, CA).

8. 5× PrimeScript®RT Master Mix (TakaRa, Dalian, China).

9. 2× SYBR Premix EX Taq II (TakaRa).

10. GlycoBlue™ Coprecipitant (Thermo Fisher).

2.2   Luciferase Reporter Assay

2.2.1   Vector Construction

1. Luciferase reporter vector: pGL3 control vector (Promega) is used as a firefly luciferase reporter vector. Putative circular RNA sequences are cloned downstream of the firefly luciferase gene in the 3′-UTR.

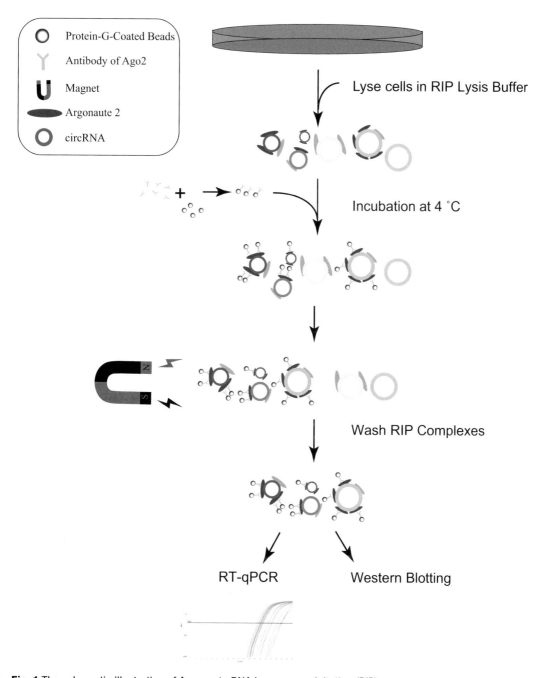

Fig. 1 The schematic illustration of Argonaute RNA immunoprecipitation (RIP) assay

2. pRL-CMV Renilla luciferase reporter (Promega): pRL-CMV is used as a Renilla luciferase control reporter vector.

3. PrimerSTAR Max DNA Polymerase Mix (Takara Bio Inc.).

2.2.2 Cell Culture   1. HEK-293T cells (American Type Culture Collection, ATCC) (*see* **Note 1**).

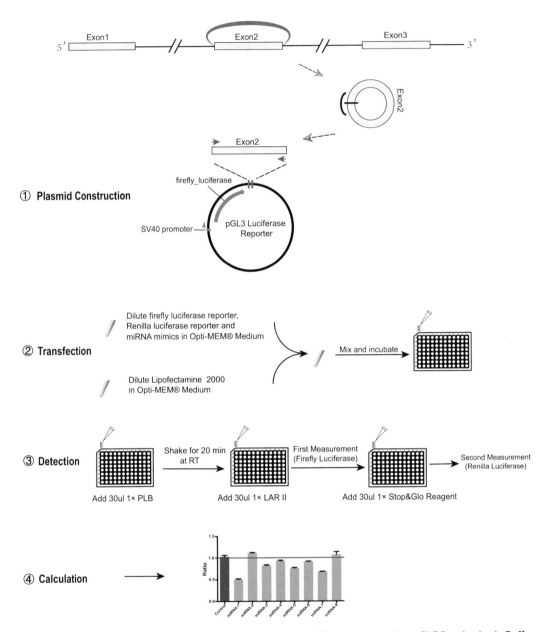

Fig. 2 The schematic illustration of luciferase screening assay. *RT* room temperature, *PLB* Passive Lysis Buffer, *LAR II* luciferase assay reagent II

2. 1× Trypsin-EDTA solution.

3. Fetal bovine serum (FBS) sterile.

4. Dulbecco's modified Eagle medium (DMEM) supplemented with antibiotics and 10% FBS.

5. Antibiotics: Penicillin (100 U/mL)/streptomycin (100 μg/mL).

2.2.3 Transfection	1. Opti-MEM® I Reduced Serum Medium (Gibco).
	2. Transfection reagent Lipofectamine 2000 (Invitrogen).
	3. miRNA mimics (*see* **Note 2**).
	4. 96-Well plate, white, flat bottom, with lid (plate for luminescence).
2.2.4 Luciferase Measurement	1. Passive Lysis Buffer (Dual Luciferase System, Promega).
	2. Luciferase Assay Reagent II (LAR II): Luciferase Assay.
	3. Substrate, and Luciferase Assay Buffer II (Dual Luciferase System, Promega).
	4. Stop & Glo Reagent: Stop & Glo Buffer and 50× Stop & Glo Substrate (Dual Luciferase System, Promega).
	5. Luminometer.

3 Methods

3.1 AGO2 RNA Immunoprecipitation	1. Wash cells twice with 1× ice-cold PBS, then add 3 mL PBS, scrape cells carefully on ice, and harvest cells by centrifugation at $800 \times g$ for 5 min at 4 °C (approximately 1×10^7 cells) (*see* **Note 3**).
3.1.1 Lysate Preparation	2. Discard the supernatant, add 300 µL RIP ice-cold lysis buffer and 1 µL RNase Inhibitor, gently mix cells until no lumps, and incubate for 30 min on ice.
	3. Store at −80 °C.
3.1.2 Prepared Immune-Magnetic Beads	1. Add 50 µL protein-G-coated magnetic beads per tube, wash twice with 500 µL RIP ice-cold lysis buffer, and resuspend the magnetic beads with 100 µL RIP ice-cold lysis buffer (*see* **Notes 4** and **5**).
	2. Add 4 µg of the antibody of Ago2, rotating the incubation at room temperature for 30 min to allow the binding of antibody to coated beads.
	3. Centrifuge the tube at $1000 \times g$ for 15 s before the tube is placed in a magnetic field, and remove the supernatant.
	4. Wash the beads twice with 500 µL RIP ice-cold lysis buffer, resuspend the magnetic beads with 500 µL RIP ice-cold lysis buffer, and place on ice.
3.1.3 Immunoprecipitation of Protein-RNA Complexes	1. Add 2 µL RNA inhibitor into 700 µL ice-cold lysis buffer to prepare precipitation buffer.
	2. Put the magnetic beads (from **step 4** in Subheading 3.1.2) in magnetic field, remove the supernatant, and resuspend it with precipitation buffer.

3. Centrifuge the cell lysate (**step 3** in Subheading 3.1.1) at 14,000 × g for 10 min at 4 °C, divert 100 µL of supernatant to each antibody-bead reaction, and incubate the tube on rotating wheel overnight at 4 °C.

4. Take 5 µL (5%) of the cell lysate, place it in two new tubes labeled "Input", and store at −80 °C.

5. After the overnight incubation, centrifuge the antibody-bead tube, place it in a magnetic field, and remove the supernatant.

6. Add 500 µL of ice-cold lysis buffer to the tube, mix it gently, incubate for 1 min, place it in magnetic field, and discard the supernatant.

7. Repeat step 6 another four times with 500 µL of ice-cold lysis buffer.

8. Take 20% of step 7 into a new tube, place them in magnetic field, and discard the supernatant.

9. Add 30 µL 1× protein SDS-PAGE loading buffer into a tube of 5% "Input" (**step 4** in Subheading 3.1.3) and the sample (**step 8** in Subheading 3.1.3), and incubate at 100 °C for 15 min, used for test precipitation efficiency by western blotting.

3.1.4 RNA Purification

1. Add 1 mL TRIzol into another tube of 5% "Input" and the rest 80% of **step 8** in Subheading 3.1.3, mix by pipetting, and incubate at room temperature for 5 min.

2. Add 200 µL chloroform and vortex the samples vigorously.

3. Centrifuge the tubes at 12,000 × g for 15 min at 4 °C, divert 400 µL of supernatant to a new tube, and add an equal volume of isopropanol and 1 µL glycogen into every tube.

4. Centrifuge the tubes at 12,000 × g for 10 min at 4 °C, and discard the supernatant.

5. Add 1 mL 75% ice-cold ethanol, and centrifuge at 7500 × g for 5 min at 4 °C.

6. Discard the supernatant, and air-dry the tubes.

7. Resuspend the tubes in 20 µL of RNase-free water, incubate for 10 min at 65 °C, and place them on ice.

8. Reverse transcript the equal volume of RNA with 5× PrimeScript®RT Master Mix for quantitative detection.

3.1.5 Quantitative Real-Time PCR Analysis

1. Reaction system:

2× SYBR Premix	5 µL.
50× ROX	0.2 µL.
Primers (forward and reverse)	1 µL (5 pmol each).
Template	3.8 µL.

Cover the platform with MicroAmp, and centrifuge at 1000 × g for 1 min.

Amplification system:

Denaturation for 15 s at 95 °C; and 5 s at 95 °C; then 30 s at 60 °C, total 40 cycles.

2. Check the melt curve to confirm that each reaction produces a single specific product.

3. Export all result with appropriate labels in an Excel spreadsheet.

4. Calculate the average Ct of 5% Input as internal reference:

ΔCt = Ct (Ago2 or IgG)—Average Ct (5% Input).

5. Calculate RIP fold enrichment above the 5% Input:

Fold enrichment = $2^{-\Delta Ct}$

3.2 Luciferase Reporter Assay (See Note 6)

1. The genomic region for circular RNA is obtained in the website of UCSC (http://genome.ucsc.edu) or circBase (http://www.circbase.org) (*see* **Note** 7).

3.2.1 Vector Construction

2. PCR amplification of the circular RNA sequence using PrimerSTAR Max DNA Polymerase Mix (Takara Bio Inc.).

3. Luciferase reporter vector linearization and PCR fragment digestion.

4. Agarose gel is retrieved to purify both linearized vector and digested PCR fragment.

5. Combine the vector with the appropriate purified PCR fragment.

6. Add the ligation product to DH5α bacterial competent cells.

7. Incubate the transformed cells at 37 °C on LB agar plates with 100 μg/mL of ampicillin overnight.

8. Inoculate LB medium with 100 μg/mL ampicillin with isolated clones at 37 °C with shaking overnight.

9. Purify plasmid DNA using the plasmid preparation kit according to the manufacturer's instructions.

10. All constructs were verified by sequencing.

3.2.2 Transfection

1. Discard the cell culture medium and wash with PBS.

2. Detach adherent cells by trypsinization.

3. Resuspend the cells with complete DMEM medium. For transfection in 96-well plates seed 5000 HEK-293 T cells per well in 100 μL media. Keep the cells at 37 °C and 5% CO_2 for 12–24 h.

4. According to the manufacturer's instructions, HEK-293 T cells were transfected with a mixture of 50 ng firefly luciferase reporter, 5 ng pRL-CMV Renilla luciferase reporter, and 5 pmol miRNA mimics per well using Lipofectamine 2000, in

a final volume of 15 μL Opti-MEM I Reduced Serum Medium per well. Perform each reaction mix in triplicate.

5. Incubate for 5 min at room temperature.

6. Meanwhile, prepare 0.25 μL of Lipofectamine 2000 and 15 μL of Opti-MEM I Reduced Serum Medium per well. Mix by pipetting up and down several times.

7. Incubate for 5 min at room temperature.

8. Add the Lipofectamine 2000 mixture on the plasmid mixture and mix thoroughly.

9. Incubate at room temperature for 20 min.

10. Add the 30 μL transfection mixture drop by drop to the cells.

11. Incubate cells for 48 h at 37 °C with 5% CO_2.

3.2.3 The Detection of Luciferase Activities

1. After 48 h, discard the culture medium and wash the cells with 1× PBS buffer.

2. Add 30 μL of 1× Passive Lysis Buffer to each well.

3. Gently shake the 96-well plates at room temperature for 20 min.

4. Prepare a sufficient amount of LAR II Buffer (firefly luciferase substrate) and Stop & Glo buffer (firefly luciferase inhibitor and Renilla luciferase substrate). For each well, prepare 30 μL of LARII Buffer and 30 μL of Stop & Glo buffer. Thaw in bath at room temperature and mix gently by inverting the vial several times before using.

5. Add 30 μL LAR II Buffer to each culture well. Place the plate in the luminometer to measure the firefly luciferase activity.

6. Add 30 μL Stop & Glo buffer to each culture well. Place the plate in the luminometer to measure the Renilla luciferase activity.

7. For each experiment, calculate the relative luciferase activities compared with control. The ratio of firefly luciferase activity/Renilla luciferase activity is used to normalize luciferase activity (*see* **Notes 8** and **9**).

4   Notes

1. HEK-293 T cells were used in this assay due to the high transfection efficiency. Other comparable cell lines can also be chosen and the efficiency of the transfection needs to be optimized.

2. Use TargetScan program (http://www.targetscan.org/vert_61/) to predict the miRNAs binding to circRNA sequence. This analysis has to be performed in local computer because the TargetScan website only provides the analysis of UTR sequences.

3. The preventive measure on working with AGO2 RIP is to use water, instruments, tips, and tubes RNase free. Gloves and pipettes may be accurately new before the use.

4. The type of beads utilized for the immunoprecipitation should depend on the type of the antibody of Argonaute2. Mouse and rabbit monoclonal antibodies both have stronger affinity for protein G. Therefore, preparing protein G-coated magnetic beads is appropriate.

5. To remove the supernatant, place the tubes in the magnetic support and wait for the complete settling of beads on the tube site that interact with the magnet. While aspirating the supernatant, be sure to change tips between the samples. Resuspending the complex of beads and RIP lysis buffer needs to be gentle, avoiding having the bubble.

6. If the circRNA was specifically enriched from Ago2 RIP assay, this result suggests that some miRNAs may bind to the circRNA. Then we can use the TargetScan prediction program to find miRNA-binding sites in the circRNA region. Combined with the expression of these miRNAs in some databases, such as TCGA, we can identify some candidate miRNAs to perform the next luciferase reporter assay.

7. The fragment we amplified is linear; however, circRNA is covalently closed noncolinear RNA, so the miRNA-binding sites in the junction site of circRNA are not considered in this experiment.

8. If the luciferase reporter activity is significantly reduced, we can then mutate each miRNA target site from the luciferase reporter to investigate the specific binding sites.

9. To distinguish miRNA sponge or miRNA targeting, the miRNA mimic may transfect into the cells and examine the expression level of circRNA. If the expression level of circRNA was not significantly changed by miRNA, the circRNA may function as a sponge to this miRNA. If the expression level of circRNA was downregulated by miRNA, the circRNA may be a target of miRNA.

Acknowledgments

This work was supported by grants from the National Natural Science Foundation of China (81672779, 81502430, and 81472617).

References

1. Glazar P, Papavasileiou P, Rajewsky N (2014) circBase: a database for circular RNAs. RNA 20:1666–1670

2. Guo JU, Agarwal V, Guo H, Bartel DP (2014) Expanded identification and characterization of mammalian circular RNAs. Genome Biol 15:409

3. You X, Vlatkovic I, Babic A, Will T, Epstein I, Tushev G et al (2015) Neural circular RNAs are derived from synaptic genes and regulated by development and plasticity. Nat Neurosci 18:603–610

4. Rybak-Wolf A, Stottmeister C, Glazar P, Jens M, Pino N, Giusti S et al (2015) Circular RNAs in the mammalian brain are highly abundant, conserved, and dynamically expressed. Mol Cell 58:870–885

5. Burd CE, Jeck WR, Liu Y, Sanoff HK, Wang Z, Sharpless NE (2010) Expression of linear and novel circular forms of an INK4/ARF-associated non-coding RNA correlates with atherosclerosis risk. PLoS Genet 6:e1001233

6. Geng HH, Li R, YM S, Xiao J, Pan M, Cai XX et al (2016) The circular RNA Cdr1as promotes myocardial infarction by mediating the regulation of miR-7a on its target genes expression. PLoS One 11:e0151753

7. WW D, Yang W, Chen Y, ZK W, Foster FS, Yang Z et al (2017) Foxo3 circular RNA promotes cardiac senescence by modulating multiple factors associated with stress and senescence responses. Eur Heart J 38:1402–1412

8. Yang W, WW D, Li X, Yee AJ, Yang BB (2016) Foxo3 activity promoted by non-coding effects of circular RNA and Foxo3 pseudogene in the inhibition of tumor growth and angiogenesis. Oncogene 35:3919–3931

9. Guarnerio J, Bezzi M, Jeong JC, Paffenholz SV, Berry K, Naldini MM et al (2016) Oncogenic role of fusion-circRNAs derived from cancer-associated chromosomal translocations. Cell 165:289–302

10. Huang G, Zhu H, Shi Y, Wu W, Cai H, Chen X (2015) cir-ITCH plays an inhibitory role in colorectal cancer by regulating the Wnt/beta-catenin pathway. PLoS One 10:e0131225

11. Li Z, Huang C, Bao C, Chen L, Lin M, Wang X et al (2015) Exon-intron circular RNAs regulate transcription in the nucleus. Nat Struct Mol Biol 22:256–264

12. Zhang Y, Zhang XO, Chen T, Xiang JF, Yin QF, Xing YH et al (2013) Circular intronic long noncoding RNAs. Mol Cell 51:792–806

13. Hansen TB, Jensen TI, Clausen BH, Bramsen JB, Finsen B, Damgaard CK et al (2013) Natural RNA circles function as efficient microRNA sponges. Nature 495:384–388

14. Memczak S, Jens M, Elefsinioti A, Torti F, Krueger J, Rybak A et al (2013) Circular RNAs are a large class of animal RNAs with regulatory potency. Nature 495:333–338

15. Conn SJ, Pillman KA, Toubia J, Conn VM, Salmanidis M, Phillips CA et al (2015) The RNA binding protein quaking regulates formation of circRNAs. Cell 160:1125–1134

16. Zheng Q, Bao C, Guo W, Li S, Chen J, Chen B et al (2016) Circular RNA profiling reveals an abundant circHIPK3 that regulates cell growth by sponging multiple miRNAs. Nat Commun 7:11215

17. Hansen TB, Wiklund ED, Bramsen JB, Villadsen SB, Statham AL, Clark SJ et al (2011) miRNA-dependent gene silencing involving Ago2-mediated cleavage of a circular antisense RNA. EMBO J 30:4414–4422

INDEX

Christoph Dieterich and Argyris Papantonis (eds.), *Circular RNAs: Methods and Protocols*, Methods in Molecular Biology,
vol. 1724, https://doi.org/10.1007/978-1-4939-7562-4, © Springer Science+Business Media, LLC 2018

Printed in the United States
By Bookmasters